Regina Holze
Speech Acts in Securitization

Culture and Language | 4

Regina Holze, born in 1992, works at Europa-Universität Flensburg. Prior to this, she completed her PhD and taught at Universität Passau in the field of political linguistics. In addition to political language and pandemic crisis communication, her research focuses on innovative approaches and digital elements in higher education pedagogy.

Regina Holze

Speech Acts in Securitization

Strategies in British Government Communication in the COVID-19 Pandemic

[transcript]

Doctoral thesis, submitted to the University of Passau

Bibliographic information published by the Deutsche Nationalbibliothek
The Deutsche Nationalbibliothek lists this publication in the Deutsche Nationalbibliografie; detailed bibliographic data are available online at https://dnb.dnb.de

Hermannstraße 26 | D-33602 Bielefeld | live@transcript-verlag.de

Cover design: Maria Arndt
Cover illustration: photo by Bernd Dittrich (@hdbernd) / Unsplash, 2023
Printing: Elanders Waiblingen GmbH, Waiblingen
https://doi.org/10.14361/9783839480250
Print-ISBN: 978-3-8376-8423-0 | PDF-ISBN: 978-3-8394-8025-0
ISSN of series: 2944-5310 | eISSN of series: 2944-5329

Printed on permanent acid-free text paper.

Für Hann und meine Mama, die mich jeden einzelnen Tag liebevoll unterstützen und an mich glauben.

Contents

Acknowledgment

Diese Arbeit ist das Ergebnis von vier Jahren intensiver Auseinandersetzung mit Sprache, Daten und Pandemiegeschehen. Sie ist ohne die Unterstützung zahlreicher Menschen nicht denkbar. Deshalb möchte ich an dieser Stelle ganz herzlich danken:

- meiner Doktormutter, Professorin Dr. Daniela Wawra von der Universität Passau, die mir die Chance gegeben hat, mich in einen neuen Themenbereich einzuarbeiten und die mich jahrelang geduldig begleitet, in die richtige Richtung geleitet und motiviert hat. Es gab keine Besprechung, aus der ich nicht voller Elan gekommen wäre. Danke Daniela!
- meiner Zweitgutachterin, PD Dr. Helene Schmolz, für ihre Zeit, ihre sorgfältige Lektüre und ihre wertvollen Hinweise, wo Präzisierungen und Nachschärfungen nötig waren.
- der anonymen Reviewperson des transcript Verlags, die mir neben pointierten und konstruktiven Anmerkungen auch das wunderbare Kompliment hinterlassen hat, eine versierte Analytikerin zu sein.
- Boris Johnson, dem ehemaligen britischen Premier, für seine rhetorische Kreativität und Selbstsicherheit, die diese Arbeit inhaltlich bereichern und für Unterhaltung beim Schreiben gesorgt haben.
- dem Frauenbüro der Universität Passau, heute Stabsstelle Diversity und Gleichstellung, allen voran Antje Sarodnik, für das Stipendium, das mir Freiraum und vor allem Schreibzeit verschafft hat.
- meinen ehemaligen Kolleg*innen und jetzigen Freund*innen von der Uni Passau. Aus tiefstem Herzen Danke für eure liebevolle Unterstützung, eure unermüdliche Hilfsbereitschaft und die vielen Gespräche von der ersten Idee bis zur letzten Fußnote. Was für ein wilder Ritt! Julia, Flo, Petra, Amelie, Viola – ihr seid toll!

- meiner Tochter, die mir den nötigen Ansporn gegeben hat, diese Arbeit fertigzustellen, um endlich entspannt auf den Spielplatz gehen zu können – und meiner Mama, die sie so oft liebevoll betreut hat, um mir Zeit zum Schreiben zu ermöglichen.
- und ganz besonders meinem wunderbaren Mann, der mich jeden Tag motiviert, unterstützt, mit Kaffee versorgt, bekocht und dafür sorgt, dass ich den Kopf nicht in den Sand stecke. Er musste sich unzählige Male spätnachts über Korpora und Statistik unterhalten und hat stets bemerkenswerte Geduld bewiesen. Ohne dich hätte der Vogel Strauß wohl gewonnen. DANKE!

1 Introduction

The virus SARS-CoV-2, also known as the coronavirus or COVID-19[1], and its impact on everyday life have had a profound effect on the global socio-political and communicative landscape since early 2020. The pandemic's far-reaching implications for public health, economic stability and daily life challenged governments worldwide to engage in complex decision-making processes in order to balance the medical, economic and social well-being of their citizens. In many cases, this balancing act led to the imposition of restrictions on public life as the risks posed by the virus were deemed to outweigh the negative consequences of such measures.

The societal impact of the pandemic has been profound, resulting in the disruption of established norms as well as the politicisation of the situation on a global scale. The response of governments varied greatly, with some countries, such as Brazil and Sweden, opting for minimal interventions, while others, including New Zealand and Vietnam, implemented strict lockdowns. Marsen and Ali-Chand (2022: 19) posit that these differing approaches not only reflect the divergent socio-economic policies of the respective governments but also highlight their distinct communication strategies, which aim to frame the crisis, manage public perception and foster compliance. In this context, language functions as a key tool for the construction, legitimisation and dissemination of these approaches, thereby exposing the inherent interdependence between political crisis management and communication.

Simultaneously, communication in the form of governmental press conferences became a central feature of public life during the pandemic (cf. Allen et al. 2024: 751; Schueler and Marx 2023: 870). With alternative forms of social interaction severely restricted, these televised addresses transcended their

---

1 For consistency and better readability, the virus will be called 'COVID-19' in the following.

traditional role as channels for the dissemination of information. Instead, they evolved into collective "event[s]" (Hayek 2024: 1), uniting audiences in their shared anticipation of rising or falling infection rates, eased restrictions or new developments. For many, these press conferences represented a break from the monotony of lockdown life, offering both clarity and a shared space for collective reflection during a time of uncertainty (cf. Dau and Ellis 2023: 34f.; Hayek 2024: 2).

This study conducts a corpus-based discourse analysis of governmental communication during the COVID-19 pandemic. It focuses on the speech acts employed in official press statements by the British government during the initial phase of the crisis. In examining the securitizing function of these speech acts by the UK[2] head of government, Prime Minister Boris Johnson, this research aims to shed light on the speech acts that shape public perception and response during an unprecedented global crisis. The empirical findings are then aggregated to determine the general structure of speech acts over the length of the securitizing statement.

The dissertation commences with a comprehensive outline of the theoretical foundations of the analysis. It begins with a **theoretical introduction** to speech act theory, as originally developed by Austin (1962) and further refined by Searle (1969). This is followed by a detailed discussion of securitization theory, as conceptualised by Buzan, Wæver and de Wilde (1998), which provides the framework for understanding how linguistic constructions shape perceptions of security threats. **Chapter three** bridges the gap between these theoretical approaches by exploring the connection between speech acts and securitization. In **chapter four**, the research design is introduced, beginning with the identification of a notable research gap in the lack of a pragmatic

2 The term 'Great Britain' is primarily used geographically, denoting the island that comprises England, Scotland, and Wales as well as the associated isles. In contrast, the name 'United Kingdom' designates the independent country, encompassing Great Britain and Northern Ireland, in a purely political sense (cf. Cunningham 2018: 1). This study focuses on the communication by British Prime Minister Johnson regarding the COVID-19 pandemic. Even though he comments on a topic related to health, which is among the responsibilities of the devolved authorities of the four nations within the United Kingdom, and most of his announced measures consequently pertain solely to England (cf. Paun et al. 2020: 1), he is speaking for the whole country in his capacity as prime minister. Therefore, the term 'United Kingdom', or its abbreviation 'UK', is employed throughout this work.

approach to the securitization process, which would significantly aid in understanding the ways in which utterances contribute to the linguistic construction of security threats. It continues with the formulation of two research questions and proceeds to provide a detailed description of the selected methodology for this work, corpus-assisted discourse analysis. Following a discussion of the criteria for compiling corpora, these are then applied in order to construct the research corpus consisting of British government press statements. The study then introduces corpus-assisted discourse analysis as a methodological approach, providing a detailed discussion of the advantages of combining the two approaches critical discourse analysis and corpus linguistics. The subsequent **chapter five** constitutes the primary empirical analysis, focusing on a case study of the securitizing speech acts used by the United Kingdom's Prime Minister Boris Johnson during the pandemic. It begins with a description of the securitization events in Great Britain during 2020, followed by a description of the corpus and an initial examination with corpus analysis methods. Afterwards, the individual speech acts employed in this securitizing move are analysed across the five speech act categories, which culminates in a meta-analysis of speech act distribution patterns and recurring co-occurrences of categories. **Chapter six** synthesises and abstracts the findings in order to answer the two research questions. First, it outlines all speech acts present in this corpus of securitizing press statements. Building on these, it seeks to define a prototypical structure for speech acts used in securitizing moves during crises. The study **concludes** with a discussion of potential future research directions in the fields of speech act analysis, securitization theory and crisis communication.

2 Theory

This study explores the relationship between *Speech Act Theory*, a linguistic theory, and the concept of *Securitization*, an established framework in the field of politics. *Securitization*[1] describes the process of ascribing urgency and importance to a particular political issue, framing it as a potentially existential threat to a nation or group. The objective is to convince the potentially affected group of the presented interpretation of the situation. If successful, it results in a demand for the immediate implementation of urgent and far-reaching emergency measures in order to resolve the issue. Language in the form of speech acts is the central element in these deliberations as it is the instrument through which the success of a securitization attempt is decided. Speech acts are an integral part of the securitizing process.

Both theories place significant emphasis on the performative capacity of language to influence reality. They describe how language is able to perform actions that extend beyond the mere transmission of information when used in a suitable context. This relationship between language and action constitutes the subject of this study. In order to achieve a deeper understanding of the underlying assumptions and implications of these two theories, a detailed examination will be conducted, commencing with a comprehensive overview of speech act theory and followed by an examination of securitization.

1 In this study, the term 'securitization' is spelled with a 'z', despite otherwise adhering to British English conventions. This spelling originates from the original framework by Buzan, Wæver, and de Wilde (1998) and is retained as a technical term. Consequently, all inflected forms, such as 'securitizing', follow this spelling.

2.1 Speech Act Theory

2.1.1 Core assumptions of Speech Act Theory

Speaking any language involves behaving in certain rule-governed ways, as Searle stated over 50 years ago (cf. 1969: 16). Meaningful communication is not only ensured through the rules of a language but also through the pragmatics of its linguistic acts. However, the minimal unit for this is not merely a word or symbol, according to Searle, but rather the speech act, which refers to the "production or issuance of a sentence token under certain conditions" (Searle 1969: 16). The concept of speech acts, first mentioned in 1933 by Karl Bühler, mainly stems from John L. Austin's work. In a series of 1955 lectures at Harvard University, and in his book *How to Do Things with Words*, he elaborates his understanding of speech as action. He observes that there is one type of sentence that expresses truths or falsehoods, while a second type performs actions instead. Thus, he distinguishes between constative and performative utterances, the latter of which cannot be measured by the dichotomy of true or false, but rather in terms of success (cf. Austin 1962: 94). To evaluate this, he proposes considering the circumstances of an utterance in order to grasp its full meaning, as speaking words is just one part of performing an act. For the achievement of a desired outcome, specific predefined conditions are often necessary at the time of the utterance (cf. Austin 1962: 8f.). If these conditions are met, then saying something can simultaneously result in an action being performed. Speech act theory therefore explains how language works in the context of various communicative settings, moving the focus towards the interaction between speaker and audience. Moving "discourse from the 'statement' to the 'utterance' level, Austin explored its performative aspect, which aims to produce changes in the world, shift behaviours and attitudes, and elicit reactions" (Marsen and Ali-Chand 2022: 24). Since then, speech acts have developed into an established concept not only in linguistics but also within philosophy and other cognitive and social sciences (cf. Harris et al. 2018: 1).

2.1.2 Austin's systematic in describing speech acts

Building on this theoretical understanding of speech acts, it is essential to examine how Austin conceptualises the structure and systematic nature of speech acts. Subdividing his concept into layers, he differentiates three levels of speech act performance:

- locutionary act,
- illocutionary act, and
- perlocutionary act.

The first refers to the pure act of "uttering certain noises" (Austin 1962: 95) that belong and adhere to the grammar of a language, i.e. the act of saying something. The illocutionary act is the stage of giving meaning to these noises by performing some kind of action with them. It centres on the act of doing something by uttering something. Thirdly, perlocutionary acts encompass the effects caused by the illocutionary act on the audience, therefore referring to the consequence of the speech act (cf. Austin 1962: 108).[2]

Austin lists four **basic requirements** for the act of performing something by speaking. First, a procedure or convention must have been established among the people involved. They must agree that uttering certain words under specific circumstances has an effect beyond merely uttering morphemes (cf. Austin 1962: 14). These agreements can be established customs within a society, legal frameworks or social institutions (cf. Harris et al. 2018: 2). To be carried out effectively, these circumstances need to be present at the moment of speaking. Furthermore, the participants in the exchange need to conduct themselves in the correct and complete manner expected from them. If these criteria are not met, then the intended act cannot be achieved; it misfires. Austin calls these "purported acts" (Austin 1962: 16) or attempts. Moreover, the intended procedure often requires the participants to not only act correctly but also to have certain thoughts or feelings, as might be the case in, e.g. praying, condoling or betting. To perform the act, the speaker must feel or think in a corresponding way, intend to behave accordingly and then actually do so. The act itself can seemingly be achieved without this internal attitude, although it then proves void without a sincere intention behind (cf. ibid.: 14f.). Borrowing the Gricean term of felicity (cf. Grice 1975: 52ff.), Austin calls infelicitous acts

2 There are currently five theories of speech acts that focus on different elements of Austin's theory as the decisive factor in the felicity of the attempt to perform a speech act. For an elaborate discussion of the implications and challenges of conventionalism, intentionalism, functionalism, expressionism and normativism, see Harris et al. (2018).

like these "'professed' or 'hollow'" (Austin 1962: 16). One example would be the act of promising, which is generally agreed to be a binding statement of one's future behaviour. To carry out the act of promising, the person making the promise needs to be able to fulfil this action and be sincere about it, as opposed to, e.g. uttering words of promise as a joke or as part of reciting a poem. The words in the form of such a performative act can be spoken and still have an effect other than the obvious content of the utterance. 'I promise' can very well be a part of a joke or of a literary reading and be understood in this function by the audience. In this case, no actual promise is being made (cf. Austin 1962: 33). The audible utterance is therefore an outward description of the speaker's inner intention and must be interpreted by the audience in the context of the circumstances at the time of the utterance. If this inner attitude does not fulfil the sincerity criterion, the promise is still an act of promise, albeit a misleading and fraudulent one without the desired outcome, i.e. an infelicitous or unhappy performance. However, it does not become a lie or misstatement straight away as there is still a possibility of the promise being fulfilled and the act therefore being completed in the expected manner (cf. ibid.: 9ff.). Some acts, however, e.g. marrying or gifting, imply a necessity for other prerequisites, such as not already being married at the time of the wedding or being in possession of the thing one is about to gift. Due to their nature of performing an action by being uttered, Austin called them 'performative utterances'.

One type of performative utterance is **explicitly performative** due to the nature of the verb. The illocutionary force of these utterances, i.e. the intention of the speaker in producing it, is already indicated by the verb itself. It can be recognised by the real use or plausible insertion of 'hereby', e.g. in sentences such as 'hereby I baptise this ship' or 'hereby I declare war'. Additionally, they usually use the first person singular or plural, and in a few cases also a passive construct, for example, 'I hereby warn you' and 'You are hereby warned' (cf. Austin 1962: 69). These verbs are mostly used in simple present forms, in contrast to their progressive forms, which rather act as a description of the speech act. Not every verb that expresses a type of utterance can be used to construct performative speech acts in which the uttered word(s) operate(s) like the title of the attempted act. Some have a perlocutionary effect on the addressee that is not explicitly marked in the utterance. The sentence 'I hereby fire you' shows its illocutionary force directly, but 'I hereby insult you' is an uncommon utterance that is unlikely to fulfil its advertised intention and will therefore not achieve the desired effect (cf. Austin 1962: 82).

While these acts require particular words to take effect, others can also be inferred by the use of particles such as 'still', conjunctive adverbs such as 'although' or by using a particular vocal emphasis, cadence or tone. Strongly dependent on contextual cues, they implicitly suggest statements and are therefore referred to as implicit performatives (cf. ibid.: 74f.). The statement 'We are still going for a walk' in conjunction with looking out of the window can, for example, signal an acknowledgement of the fact that it is raining and of the unchanged decision to go for a walk, maybe already the call to get dressed, even if other participants of this planned walk might want to object, all without explicitly stating this. Lewis coined the term 'conversational score' to describe the insight that the qualities of a speech act shape and are shaped by their respective context and that therefore the meaning of context-specific expressions can vary considerably (cf. Lewis 1979: 345). One commonality of speech acts, however, is that they can only be performed by people. Usually, the person speaking is the performer of the act (cf. Austin 1962: 60).

2.1.3 Austin's taxonomy of speech acts

Austin tentatively differentiates five categories of illocutionary acts. The first is called '**verdictives**' and describes verbs related to stating facts or describing reasons, in the sense of giving a verdict. This assessment does not need to be final but can also express a state in an ongoing situation. Included in this class are verbs such as to acquit, to estimate, to characterise or to rank. The second category, '**exercitives**', comprises verbs expressing a decision in favour of a certain action. In contrast to verdictives, which state something, the latter make facts or shape a situation, e.g. by pleading, commanding, warning or announcing. Thirdly, '**commissives**' are committing the speaker to a certain future behaviour by declaring an intention. Verbs in this class encompass making promises, contracting or vowing, among others, but also include rather vague acts such as siding with somebody. The fourth category centres on verbs expressing a speaker's reaction to the social behaviour of others, which Austin called '**behabitives**'. Among his examples are verbs such as to congratulate, to protest, to criticise or to apologise. The last category, '**expositives**', refers to acts involved in conducting arguments, clarifying something or more generally in expounding views. Affirming, denying, answering or conceding are among the verbs listed in this fifth class, which the author himself admits is difficult to define (cf. Austin 1962: 150f.).

2.1.4 Searle's criticism of Austin

Austin's theory and especially his five categories have been refined and developed further by John Searle. He agrees with Austin that speaking "is performing speech acts, acts such as making statements, giving commands, asking questions, (...) and, secondly, that these acts are in general made possible by and are performed in accordance with certain rules for the use of linguistic elements" (Searle 1969: 16). He also concurs that there is a series of analytical links between the intention of a speaker, the meaning of their utterance, the understanding of the receiving audience and the linguistic rules governing the interaction (cf. ibid.: 21). In particular, he pays attention to indirect speech acts, where degrees of implication act as promise, direction or commission, without making an outright statement. In some cultural contexts, indirectness has been found to be related to politeness (cf. Brown and Levinson 1987; Sifianou 2012).

Austin's differentiation between locutionary, illocutionary and perlocutionary acts is met with Searle's disapproval as he argues for a finer distinction. The locutionary act, the pure action of uttering morphemes that form words and sentences, is instead called an '**utterance act**' in the latter's work *Speech Acts* (1969). Simply uttering strings of words is presented as sufficient to constitute an utterance act, just as in Austin's locutionary act. Searle's second element is termed the '**propositional act**'. It involves a reference to someone or something and the predication, i.e. the characteristics of said referent object. "A proposition is what is asserted in the act of asserting, what is stated in the act of stating" (Searle 1969: 29). It consists of "singular definite referring expressions" (Searle 1969: 26) that identify an entity or object, about which the speaker adds information or asks a question, and predications, which are the information itself. They take the grammatical form of parts of sentences, with grammatical predicates forming the predication and pronouns, proper nouns or other noun phrases building the reference. It is impossible to perform a propositional act on its own, i.e. without an illocutionary act. The third element, called '**illocutionary act**' by Searle, refers to the performativity of certain verbs in Austin's sense of doing something by saying something. Here, Searle builds on Frege's notion of linguistic correlation (cf. Frege 1984: x, §106f.) in the sense that words only have reference in the context of a sentence. The performance of the illocutionary act only takes effect via the grammatical context of a complete sentence. Both illocutionary and propositional acts consist of words in certain contexts, under particular conditions and with specific intention.

Linguistic devices indicating illocutionary force include elements like "word order, stress, intonation contour, punctuation, the mood of the verb, and the so-called performative verbs" (Searle 1969: 30). The latter can be explicit, in sentences such as 'I apologise', or be implicitly denoted by the context. In general, the circumstances of an utterance are necessary to classify its intention, especially social habits or rules on which the expression depends. It is possible to perform an utterance act without performing propositional and illocutionary acts at the same time, just as the act of ticking a box may or may not perform the act of voting, depending on specific circumstances. Even different speakers using the same morphemes, i.e. performing the same utterance act, can still be making two different statements if their propositional and illocutionary acts differ. This is again dependent on the context (cf. Searle 1969: 23ff.). To give but one example, the brother of a recently baptised child enacting the same ritual with his younger sibling will not see the same effect as the priest performing this act. However, in "performing an illocutionary act one characteristically performs propositional acts and utterance acts" (Searle 1969: 24). Exceptions are rare, e.g. brief expressions like shouting in pain, which do not have a propositional content but do exhibit an utterance act and an illocutionary act.

2.1.5 Searle's systematic in describing speech acts

Just as with Austin's differentiation between locutionary, illocutionary and perlocutionary acts, Searle disagrees with his approach to creating speech act classes. In particular, the lists with verbs that Austin provided in his taxonomy of speech act categories elicit Searle's criticism, given the former's insistence on the importance of context. Some verbs, such as 'to announce', can stand for a multitude of intentions and therefore lead to several illocutionary acts, depending on their context and, in this case, on the object that is announced. The verb only denotes the manner in which this act is performed, rather than its type, which would instead be a report, order or similar. Searle thus argues that the distinction between illocutionary act and illocutionary verbs is continuously blurred as there are only a few verbs with only one connected illocutionary act, whereas many carry the potential for different illocutionary forces (cf. Searle 1969: 9). Moreover, he finds Austin's taxonomy inconsistent and ambiguous. The principles for distinguishing these categories shift the focus from the speaker to the audience and their intentions, and even include normative approaches. This results in unclear characterisations of the five classes, where verbs might belong to several of them at the same time. Even the verbs listed as examples do not always fulfil the criteria, which further complicates the suggestive association of other similar verbs that Austin intended (cf. Searle 2012: 9ff.).

Searle therefore proposes a refined classification of speech acts based primarily on three criteria:

- illocutionary point,
- direction of fit, and
- expressed psychological state.

'**Illocutionary point**', the first criterion, refers to a speaker's primary intention in performing the speech act. For an order, this would therefore be the attempt to get the audience to do something; for a promise, it would be to commit themselves to doing something in the future. This dimension focuses on the speaker and their purpose in performing the speech act. The second criterion is called '**direction of fit**'. It centres around the question of whether the condition of the world already matches the words of the speech act or needs to change. An order or promise requires a change in the world for the speech act to be satisfied, for example. Only after the audience fulfils the action ordered is the speech act satisfied, whereas in the case of a 'promise' speech act, the speaker must personally follow through with the stated action. These two examples' direction of fit is therefore world-to-word. A description reverses this focus to word-to-world, e.g. it describes a situation as it is at present. '**Expressed psychological state**' is the last dimension in Searle's classification of speech acts. Closely related to sincerity conditions, it examines whether the speaker possesses the psychological state that they express in the performance of the speech act. Giving an order would signify an expression of desire, making a promise an expression of intention and describing something an expression of belief (cf. Hanks 2018: 123f.).

2.1.6 Searle's taxonomy of speech acts

Adhering to the three criteria described above, Searle arrives at a speech act taxonomy with five categories. Even though this matches Austin's number of categories, the terminology and classification differ significantly.

The first category encompasses verbs with an illocutionary point that states facts or information or expresses knowledge or beliefs. Called '**assertives**', their purpose is to communicate truths and commit the speaker to factual statements about the world. They are not limited to true or positive statements but also encompass illocutionary acts of finding something false or wrong. Thus, these illocutions can be assessed for their truthfulness, with their direction of fit following word-to-world (cf. Searle 1976: 8ff.). The linguistic structure of sentences in this class of speech acts comprises a pronoun in the first person singular, which represents the speaker, in combination with a verb in its indicative form, followed by an optional 'that' and then the content of the statement. It is expressed as "I verb (that) + S" (Searle 1976: 17). However, this does not preclude the existence of assertive speech acts in any other form. Although often following the straightforward syntactic structure outlined here, they can also employ other subjects or follow a less schematic wording. For example, in the case of this study examining political statements, the plural pronoun 'we' being used in relation to the government might be a common occurrence. In addition, the pre-set 'I verb that' may be abbreviated, leaving only the content of the message. The assertive 'I state that' or 'I think that' is thus silently implied without naming the speech act explicitly, thereby maintaining the natural flow of language. However, these variations in expression can often be traced back to this basic form. The use of modal verbs or adverbs of certainty may further indicate the speaker's degree of confidence in the asserted proposition. Strategically, speech acts like explaining, affirming, reporting or updating also reinforce a position of authority as the speaker has the opportunity and power to guide the discourse and can carry out these acts with the expectation that the audience will listen to them. In the case of this study, the corpus includes statements such as "For 3 weeks now, the number of new cases identified through testing each day has been below 1,000[sic]" (Johnson 2020z: 1), which are pertinent to this class.

Speech acts in the second category are called '**directives**' as they involve the speaker directing the audience to do something. Their common illocutionary point is the speaker's intention to persuade somebody to perform a particular action. This can be achieved through a variety of means, ranging from a rather inviting speech act, such as suggesting politely with instances of hedging, to more authoritative ones, such as ordering or commanding. The former includes questions, which prompt the listener to answer, also a future action, or to behave in accordance with the speaker's instructions. The latter frequently employs modal auxiliaries such as 'must' and 'need to', as well as imperative forms with the propositional content that the audience should perform some kind of action in the future. Its sincerity condition is therefore a desire and the direction of fit follows the order world-to-word (cf. Searle 1976: 11). The structure of these speech acts typically comprises a pronoun in the first person singular, accompanied by a verb of desire and the object 'you' referring to the audience[3], followed by the requested action in the form of a verb phrase. This can be extended with a noun phrase or an adverb. One example sentence is 'I order you to go outside', which consists of 'I order you' + 'you will go' + 'outside'. It therefore looks like this: "I verb you + you Fut Vol Verb (NP) (Adv)" (Searle 1976: 17). As stated above in relation to assertives, directive speech acts can also use a different subject, e.g. 'we', or abbreviate this structure in various ways so that the specific name of the illocutionary verb is no longer stated. Nevertheless, the illocutionary point remains unchanged. Directives are focused on the listeners and the actions required of them, while excluding the speaker, who is not addressed in the demand for an action. In this study's corpus, one example of a directive statement is Johnson's utterance: "wash your hands with soap and hot water" (Johnson 2020a: 1).

'**Commissives**', which make up the third category, reverse this focus away from the audience to the speaker's future actions. By employing this kind of illocutionary verb, they commit themselves to doing something. Examples are to promise, to pledge or to threaten, i.e. verbs with an intention as their sincerity condition and a world-to-word direction of fit (cf. Searle 1976: 11f.). As promises are among the acts with the strongest illocutionary forces indicating a commitment, they are frequently used to emphasise one's commitment to something, even if the situation itself does not require this speech act. In such cases, the promise does not fulfil the speech act 'promise' but rather reinforces the other (cf. Searle 1969: 58f.). For example, in moments where the speaker wants to refute an allegation strongly, a promise adds emphasis to their denial. The executed speech act is then 'deny'[4], which focuses on events in the past, and not the commissive 'promise', which would relate to future actions. The speaker

3 As Streeck (1980: 139) remarks, this structure is unable to differentiate between different addressees but summarises them under the pronoun 'you'. Therefore, the interpretation of the speech act depends largely on the context and may not be clearly identifiable in some cases even though it directly addresses the addressee. Among others, Günthner (2021) and Holze (2023: 186) already commented on this specific problem within corpus linguistic analyses without providing a solution.

4 Usually read as an assertive speech act, Yassine Khaya recently proposed to understand 'deny' as a directive speech act instead (cf. Khaya 2024: 144).

thus commits to the accompanying statement but does not fulfil a commissive speech act in the sense of committing themselves to doing something in the future. The linguistic structure of this category is similar to that of directive speech acts as the only difference consists of the verb phrase subject. Commissives have the speaker themselves, i.e. 'I' or 'we', as the subject that is expected to do something: "I verb (you) + I Fut Vol Verb (NP)(Adv)" (Searle 1976: 17). An example is the sentence 'I promise to go there', which consists of 'I promise' + 'I will go' + 'there'. This can be contracted to the briefer form 'I will go there', which expresses the speaker's commitment in the same way, although without explicitly stating the act of promising. The propositional content of the phrase is always the speaker doing something. Consequently, commissive speech acts are limited to the use of pronouns in the first person, either singular or plural. One example of a commissive speech act is the utterance "we will reimburse the cost" (Johnson 2020e: 3). In the special corpus for this study, warnings constitute a particular case of commissives. While frequently understood as directives, they are considered as a subdivision of threats in this context, given that they often implicitly foreshadow punitive measures or the future escalation of restrictions in the event of non-compliance. The statement of 4 November illustrates this. After a call to adhere to the rules, he adds: "Otherwise we face a bleak and an uncertain future of steadily rising infections and admissions until as I say the capacity of the NHS is breached" (Johnson 2020am: 2). The implication of severe consequences is implied strongly. Therefore, warnings are marked under the category 'commissives', even though some of them do not adhere to the criteria of this category explained above.

The fourth class in Searle's taxonomy contains what are known as '**expressives**', speech acts which express the speaker's own feelings. These can be positive or negative, but all of them establish an emotive connection between speaker and audience. This class is united by the absence of a direction of fit. The speaker is neither attempting to make their words align with the world nor vice versa. Rather, they are expressing their feelings in relation to the situation as it is, was or will be. This feature is also reflected in the category's syntax. Expressives are typically accompanied by a gerundive nominalisation transformation of the verb in the second part of the utterance instead of using 'that' or 'to do'. Searle's example 'I apologise for stepping on your toe' is only a correct English sentence with the gerundive form, whereas the use of 'that' leads to 'I apologise that I step on your toe' and the use of the infinitive phrase leads to 'I apologise to step on your toe', which are both grammatically incorrect. In some cases, however, nominalisation can produce a correct sentence without the use of a gerundive form, e.g. 'I apologise for my behaviour'. These two examples also illustrate that the truth of the utterance's proposition is presupposed – e.g. having stepped on somebody's toe or having behaved badly – and cannot be changed by an expressive speech act, as this merely states the speaker's feelings in relation to it. The propositional content can be an action, a characteristic of somebody or something, or a fact; however, it needs to be connected to the speaker or the audience (cf. Searle 1976: 12f.). Expressive utterances are therefore indicative of an emotive connection between speaker and audience, as the speaker shares their feelings on a topic by performing this speech act. Common examples include thanking somebody, apologising or welcoming somebody. The deep structure of expressive speech acts therefore consists of the pronoun 'I' in combination with an expressive verb and the addressee as an object in the first part. This is followed by the actor of the action – 'I' or 'you' – and a verb phrase, which is usually in form of a gerundive. Thus, the structure of expressive speech acts looks like this: "I verb you + I/you VP => gerundive nom." (Searle 1976: 18). The sentence "I want to thank you, the people of this country, for the sheer grit and guts you have shown" (Johnson 2020g: 1) is an example of a nominalisation from the corpus.

Lastly, '**declaratives**' are the fifth category of speech acts. In this class, the speaker's utterance is actively changing the condition of something. The successful performance of a declarative speech act ensures that the propositional content corresponds to reality. It brings the desired status into being by declaring it to exist. Examples of this class are 'you are fired', 'I declare war' or 'I pronounce you husband and wife'. Declarations attempt to get language to match reality, with the direction of fit being word-to-world. At the same time, world-to-word is also true, as extralinguistic conditions are required to successfully perform the speech act. More precisely, they require an appropriate context and setting, namely the presence and fulfilment of institutional regulations or conditions in order to actually take effect. The speaker and the addressee(s) need to occupy particular roles within a predefined system of rules, such as the country's legislature, the church or private property regulations. If this is ensured, the status or the condition of the object is altered from the moment of utterance, simply by the fact that the declarative speech act has been performed. Declaratives may have different degrees of explicitness. While cases such as 'I declare war' are unambiguous in their intention and embody the pure form of declaring something, as they consist of 'I declare' + the declared state, e.g. 'the state of war now exists', cases such as 'you are fired' are less clear. Syntactically, they bear resemblance to the assertive class, exemplified by the construction 'I verb (NP)' (cf. Searle 1976: 20f.), e.g. 'I fire you'. However, their illocutionary point differs. The use of assertives allows the speaker to state a fact about the world, which remains unchanged by the speaker's further actions. With declaratives, the status of the audience changes in the moment the speaker utters the words. 'You are fired' therefore functions in the same way as the example of declaring war after all: 'I declare' + 'the state of your employment is finished'. The syntax for declaratives is then "I verb NP_1 + NP_1 be pred" (Searle 1967: 20), with the noun phrase (NP_1) being the declared state. The focus of these speech acts is on the near future as they institute an immediate change in status. One example of such a speech act from the corpus is the following announcement by Boris Johnson: "Pubs and bars must close, unless they are serving substantial meals" (Johnson 2020ai: 1).

It is evident that knowledge about the speaker and their relationship with the audience is beneficial for the interpretation of speech acts. Furthermore, an awareness of the situational context, the power distribution and the role that the speaker occupies in a society may assist in the assessment of the circumstances needed for successful speech acts, particularly for declaratives to take effect.

2.1.7 Criticism of Searle

This approach to speech acts by Searle, and subsequently his taxonomy of five classes of speech acts, have been the subject of criticism by some researchers in recent decades. One of the earliest critics was Jacques **Derrida**, who in his essay *Signature Event Context* (1972) challenged the theory's understanding of speech as a performative act that conveys meaning directly. Instead, he was convinced that it is rather part of the nature of language not to be able to get across its full, unambiguous meaning. One reason for this lies in the contextual circumstances of an utterance, which also make it difficult to repeat the same speech act with the same effect in a different context. Consequently, the intention of a speaker cannot be conveyed exactly and meaning needs to be deferred constantly. This concept, which Derrida terms "[d]iffférance" (1972: 325), is diametrically opposed to Austin's and Searle's assumption that direct communication and a clear identification of a speaker's intention is possible – the premise that makes their taxonomies possible in the first place. Furthermore, in contrast to their focus on spoken language, Derrida emphasised the equal significance of writing, particularly in its capacity to convey a higher level of complexity. He posited that the written word is not constrained by the limitations of place and time, and thus has the potential to transcend these boundaries, enabling a more accurate representation of the original intention. Searle's reply (1977) refuting these points of criticism as unwarranted led to the Searle-Derrida debate, a philosophic controversy about intentionality in language.

Streeck (1980), whose empirical analysis of illocutionary speech acts in natural discourse found some inconsistencies in Searle's "meta-theoretical assumptions relating to the nature of the relationship between meaning, saying, and doing" (Streeck 1980: 140), adds several critical points. His research focused on understanding social order in interactive classroom situations. In this setting, participants in the conversation need to constantly adapt to new contexts, e.g. in the form of subsequent utterances, which then require "reinterpretations of prior understandings in the light of upcoming contingencies" (Streeck 1980: 146). Consequently, it is impossible for researchers to classify speech acts unambiguously because meaning in this setting continues to be negotiated during the conversation. Streeck points out that in a dialogue, the roles of speaker and listener constantly change. The listener selects an interpretation of the speaker's illocutionary force, thereby turning the conversation in a direction that may make it difficult to identify intention and effect in speech acts. In light of this interactive process of negotiating meaning in discourse, Streeck rejects Searle's approach to studying speech acts in isolation and calls for the analysis of speech acts in discourse within a larger framework of interaction analysis (see also Love 1999; Rajagopalan 2000).

By contrast, Jürgen **Habermas** (1998) criticises the theory's strong focus on individual speech acts and suggests a more comprehensive approach that incorporates social, political and ethical dimensions. He argues that any communication is always influenced by the social structures of the respective society and their values and norms. Similarly, he emphasises the role of power and ideology in successful communication, especially in situations with asymmetrical power relations between the discourse participants, which is absent in Austin's and Searle's texts. Consequently, Habermas introduces the concept of the 'ideal speech situation', which is between equal participants who are free from coercion and have some level of mutual understanding. They can thus communicate in a meaningful way (cf. Habermas 1990: 86ff.). In addition to Searle's and Austin's rather strategic approaches to utterances, he proposes another focus on communicative action aiming to achieve consensus, a dimension that was not even mentioned in the original theories. Similarly, Habermas notes the lack of a tool to distinguish the validity of speech acts and thus develops additional dimensions to differentiate types of speech acts with regard to their truth, sincerity and normative rightness. These types extend far beyond the illocutionary acts that Searle and Austin describe. Indeed, it would appear that any normative statements of this kind were not within the scope of their theories.

Acheoah (2017), on the other hand, criticises the two elements "speaker's intention" (2017: 1) and "linguistic convention" (ibid.: 9). In his eyes, these notions lack clear definition and a comprehensive evaluation of context, which may influence the performativity of speech acts. He believes that the emphasis Searle, like Austin, puts on the significance of linguistic conventions for fulfilling speech acts comes at the expense of a broader spectrum of discourse constraints. In particular, he is concerned with unconventional verbal and nonverbal elements of communication – such as silence or music – and their effects on a conversation (cf. Acheoah 2017: 6), which are absent in the original theory of speech acts.

In *Excitable Speech* (2021 [1997]), Judith **Butler** engages with the Austinian performativity of utterances. While she acknowledges that some utterances can have an effect in the moment of their articulation, i.e. can show performativity, she agrees with Acheoah's and to a lesser extent Streeck's criticism that the original theory's framework is too narrow and fails to encompass vital discourse dimensions. In particular, she notes a lack of attention to the political dimensions of speech. Butler identifies that a failure to consider how power relations are reflected in language may lead to the neglect of the "discursive historicity of power" (Butler 2021: 50). To illustrate her point, she presents the example of racial slurs, demonstrating that language can perpetuate power and hierarchies over time in an almost imperceptible manner, even when the initial utterance was not originally perceived as offensive. This is because the offensiveness of the slur is derived from its historical context, in which powerful actors first established its derogatory and racist meaning within a cultural context; this is then repeated and reproduced. Consequently, Butler concludes that language cannot transmit meaning neutrally. Rather, meaning is culturally shaped by social norms and conventions (cf. Butler 2021: 79; for an elaboration on gender implications, see p. 83f.). In light of these indirect effects of setting a norm, Butler challenges Austin's assumption that performative acts always have a direct effect on reality, regardless of their context, and instead proposes a deconstructivist perspective. She understands language not as a static system with functionally secured meanings but rather as a versatile, subversive tool for change (cf. ibid.: 146f.). This differs from Austin and Searle's perspective on language as a formalised system with predefined effects on formulaic utterances. Consequently, Butler advocates for an expansion of their theory to include these political dimensions of speech.

Notwithstanding the above criticisms, Searle's approach to speech acts has been widely accepted in linguistics because of its clarity, systematic nature and comprehensiveness. Searle's refinement and systematisation of J. L. Austin's original theory led to a more structured framework that takes into account both speaker and audience, making it easier to understand and apply. By categorising speech acts into five main types, Searle offers a clear and comprehensive taxonomy that went beyond Austin's initial distinctions. Moreover, Searle's detailed definitions and the introduction of felicity conditions contribute to the precision and applicability of his framework in various contexts of linguistic and philosophical research. These factors result in the establishment of Searle's taxonomy as a fundamental tool for the analysis of language and ensured its widespread acceptance and use in a variety of fields. Recent works using his taxonomy encompass, among others, studies on speech acts in the EFL classroom (cf. Basra and Thoyyibah 2017; Faturrochman et al. 2021), on social media (cf. Sanaa and Kushi 2012; Fazira and Amri 2023), in films (cf. Short 2007; Ridanpää 2014; Pablos-Ortega 2020; Sartika and Irawan 2021), in sports (cf. Kretchmar 2012), in translations (cf. Muttaqin et al. 2020; Zagidullina et al. 2023; Mohammed 2023) and in law (cf. Meibauer 2022; Heidi and Setyaningsih 2024). It has been successfully applied to a wide range of objects, including political statements (cf. Dylgjeri 2017; McClaughlin et al. 2021; AlAfnan and Oshchepkova 2022; Marsen and Ali-Chand 2022).

Therefore, Searle's classification of speech acts has been selected as the reference for the speech acts in this analysis. The use of speech act theory in the context of this study to analyse utterances in the initial phase of securitization – a framework that focuses on speech acts as a form of political communication – responds to the criticism by Butler and Streeck. By extending the theory's application to encompass the political dimension, the theoretical framework not only addresses the concerns raised by these scholars but also offers a nuanced understanding of how speech acts function in a political discourse setting. This expansion of the theory serves to illuminate the complexities inherent in the intersection of language, power and ideology, and sheds light on the ways in which speech acts can shape and influence political interactions.

2.2 Securitization Theory

The concept of securitization was first introduced in 1998 by Buzan, Wæver and de Wilde. This "analytical framework" (Sjöstedt 2020: 29) encapsulates the Copenhagen School of security studies' intersubjective understanding of security. It does not aspire to formulate a classic etiological theory but rather seeks to explain empirical causal mechanisms (cf. Balzacq and Guzzini 2015: 98). Over the last 25 years, securitization has evolved into an established "analytical framework that helps to pinpoint the different steps in a security process" (Sjöstedt 2019: 29) for scholars of international security studies. Its primary objective is to outline the potential of speech acts and non-discursive practices for political agenda setting as well as "conceptualizing security as a labelling for which actors can be held responsible rather than an objective feature of threats" (Buzan et al. 1998: 212). The authors' reconceptualisation of security and the subsequent expansion of the definition led to the inclusion of other, non-military sectors as threats and of more units besides the state as the focus of analysis (cf. Sjöstedt 2019: 29). Meanwhile, the framework has been used extensively for a wide array of issues, from hostile troops and minority rights to migration, diseases, drugs, human trafficking and natural disasters (cf. Nyman 2012: 52; Christou and Adamides 2013; Léonard and Kaunert 2020; Perera and Makoni 2019).

Securitization can be understood as the **superlative of politicisation**, i.e. an intensified form of rendering an issue political and describing it as a problem that needs to be addressed with political means. However, politicisation opens up an issue for discussion and initiates the consideration of a variety of potential solutions within the established political routines and institutions. Securitization, on the other hand, and especially on an international level, "means to present the issue as urgent and existential, as so important that it should not be exposed to the normal haggling of politics but should be dealt with decisively by top leaders prior to other issues" (Buzan et al. 1998: 29). The suggested measures to contain the identified issue in this scenario are therefore beyond the scope of usual political customs. Security and threat are identified and created by the same actor in order to persuade the audience to accept them as justification for extraordinary defence measures. Thus, this process is radically constructivist in nature. The obvious question of whether the issue at hand actually poses an objective existential danger is not addressed by this framework, nor can it be answered by its methods of analysis. Rather, their focus is on the process of communication and the framing of a threat, as well as on the promotion of countermeasures. After all, securitization is always preceded by the political choice to address or ignore an issue. Sometimes this prevents legitimate threats from being addressed properly, which has been called complacency, i.e. the non-securitization of apparent threats. By contrast, the securitization of non-existent threats has been termed paranoia (cf. Buzan et al. 1998: 57). Actors need to assess in advance whether a particular issue will actually benefit from increased attention and the mobilisation of all instruments, or whether the side effects of applying a security lens would instead be detrimental (cf. Buzan et al. 1998: 29). The prediction of hypothetical events and consequences in the future, and as such the evaluation of current conditions in terms of risk, is essential for securitization. The probable development of events in the absence of extraordinary measures needs to be balanced with the supposed outcome in the case of their application (cf. Buzan et al. 1998: 32).

The authors of the securitization framework differentiate between a **narrow and a wider understanding of security**. Whereas the more traditional narrow understanding has been concerned exclusively with the issues of war and force in the form of military threats, a wider understanding seeks to keep the security agenda open to a broad variety of threat types (cf. Buzan et al. 1998: 4f.). Proponents of the former fear that greater openness in the definition of security would render the term increasingly meaningless (cf. Butler and Wolf 2019: 6; see also Ayoob 1997). The authors of the framework, however, align their deliberations with the latter approach. In line with the broader perspective advocated by the Copenhagen School in the 1990s, they adopt the second, more expansive understanding of security as the foundation for their framework, allowing for the inclusion of diverse and non-traditional threat types.

To illustrate the versatility of their approach, the authors identify and elaborate on **five exemplary sectors** – military, political, environmental, societal and economic – demonstrating that the framework is not limited to traditional military and political threats but rather extends to a broader spectrum of security concerns. These additional three fields increase the potential range of application significantly (for a detailed overview, see Nyman 2012: 55ff.). A military threat, for instance, can be constituted by the presence of tanks from foreign nations along the border of a country. The securitizing actor would present them as an invading force intending an armed offensive with the goal of depopulation (cf. Buzan et al. 1998: 51). This type of threat usually centres directly on the sovereign state as the most important referent object. In contrast, a threat pertaining to the political sector would concern a danger to sovereignty in a wider sense. This could be the case when the ideological pillars of a state, e.g. human rights or the current political system, are perceived as being under attack (cf. Buzan et al. 1998: 141). On the other hand, societal securitization is concerned with threats to the identity of a group. The referent objects in such a securitization attempt are therefore "communities which self-identify as communities based on a sense of shared identity" (Nyman 2012: 56). One possible threat is mass immigration and the subsequent perceived threat to the identity or culture of the indigenous people, as in, for example, the migration to Germany in 2015 (cf. Alexander 2024: 14ff.). However, the inverse phenomenon might also be a reason for securitization within this societal category, for example when a superordinate integration project, e.g. the European Union, is pulling citizens towards a different primary identity (cf. Buzan et al. 1998: 121). In the economic context, there is an abundance of referent objects "ranging from individuals [and single companies to](...) classes and states to the abstract and complex system of the global market itself" (ibid.: 100). The fear of being excluded from a significant new development that has the potential to impact the national economy is a prime example of an economic threat (cf. Buzan et al. 1998: 102). For instance, this can be observed in the current German discourse about hybrid and electric cars (cf. Jäger 2024: 1). Similarly, environmental securitization can take place for various reasons, many of which overlap with other sectors (cf. Buzan et al. 1998: 74). They usually concern the disruption of an ecosystem in a variety of ways, either man-made, such as the emission of greenhouse gases, or not directly linked to human activity, such as earthquakes (cf. Nyman 2012: 56). One example of an environmental threat is a pollution that could potentially harm those living near the polluted site.

Cases such as the 2010 Deepwater Horizon marine oil spill in the Gulf of Mexico have severe health consequences for those involved in cleaning shores or coming into contact with oil and can thus be regarded as an instance of an environmental securitization. However, these events also have an economic impact. In this example, the Gulf Coast's fishing and tourism industries were greatly affected for years after the spill (cf. Sumaila et al. 2012: 506). This duality allows the securitizing actor to select the approach that appears especially appropriate for their target audience. It also highlights a general characteristic of securitization as threats can in most cases be interpreted in different ways. The Deepwater Horizon incident can be categorised as an environmental threat due to its undeniable impact on the marine ecosystem. Consequently, it has been securitized in this manner. At the same time, the implications from this have severe consequences for the economy in the region, such as a decline in tourism revenue or rising unemployment. Similarly, the latter can also be interpreted as a danger to societal stability because the surge in the number of unemployed individuals translates into an unexpected strain on the respective states' welfare systems, thereby underscoring the potential dangers to societal stability. This does not pose a threat on a military level, but the potential political threat might also be addressed from a state perspective. Federal decisions and guidelines for the cleanup and other deepwater oil drilling operations have the potential to restrict the freedom of action of individual states, such as Louisiana, Florida and Mississippi. It may thus also be conceptualised as a political threat. This example demonstrates that a phenomenon can be securitized from a variety of perspectives. Consequently, the securitizing actor needs to determine which perspective will resonate most with their intended audience, thereby ensuring maximum impact and persuasion. Over the course of the securitization, however, it is a common tendency for the discourse to transition from the discussion of causes to that of effects. This shift in focus results in the issue being moved from its original sphere into other sectors, e.g. through an increased emphasis on financial consequences or on social dissatisfaction with the countermeasures. This decision for a narrative is typically contested by the various actors involved, each of whom "vie[s] for primacy" (Buzan et al. 1998: 176; see also Butler and Wolf 2019: 14f.) regarding their specific threat narrative. In certain instances, different sectors may complement each other, with the magnitude of the threat being amplified when it is paired with an adjacent – concurrent or prior – conflict or problem. In other cases, however, they compete to be the dominant threat narrative in a way that erases the other perspective almost completely, e.g. in situations where the emergency demands of two simultaneous issues are antagonistic. Such a dilemma can be found in the relationship between Estonia and Russia, for example, where demands for more rights for the Russian(-speaking) minority and military concerns about Russia's influence on Estonian politics and society compete for attention. The implementation of countermeasures in response to either issue exacerbates the other, creating an intractable situation. Consequently, by framing an issue as a security threat, sectors may overlap and encroach upon each other in discourse, especially over time (cf. Buzan et al. 1998: 170).

Depending on the specific threat and its context, each securitization attempt will unequivocally look different. Nonetheless, a set of "essential qualitative features" (Balzacq 2015: 103) have been identified that constitute an ideal type of securitization. In his 2015 meta-study, Balzacq found several **charac-**

teristic features of securitization attempts mentioned in recent literature. According to his analysis, a securitization attempt needs to have a "referent object, existence, audience, securitizing moves, context, [and] exceptional measures" (Balzacq 2015: 105). The act itself is divided into three phases: the securitizing move, emergency action and desecuritization. The first of these refers to the process of an actor trying to present an issue as an existential threat to a referent object that requires the audience's full attention and immediate action. The actor does this by using speech acts to convince the audience (cf. section 2.2.4), which can then decide to ignore or modify this narrative. If they accept it, then the proposed emergency measures are likely to be implemented to avoid the predicted disaster. This initiates the second phase of securitization: emergency action. Here, the employed means far exceed those of conventional political processes and institutionalised procedures in order to address and resolve, or at least mitigate, the grave threat. The usual rules and practices no longer apply at this stage. Desecuritization denotes the concluding third phase, in which the threat is no longer existential but has become manageable or is already contained. The verbal alarmism of the earlier phases rapidly decreases, while the emergency measures are either in the process of being institutionalised or ordinary proceedings are being re-established. In some cases, it can also mean that the alleged threat is in the process of being re-categorised as belonging to other fields that are already equipped to deal with the issue, e.g. a political threat being re-categorised as a trade issue (cf. Nyman 2012: 58). There are several key conditions that are recognised as making a successful securitization more likely. Firstly, the nature of the alleged threat must be taken into consideration. Secondly, the securitizing actor needs to have a certain position of authority in order to achieve an audience's acceptance (cf. Nyman 2012: 54). Lastly, the speech act itself needs to follow the "'grammar of security' emphasizing priority, urgency and survival[sic]" (Nyman 2012: 54). In the following, these different elements of a securitization are examined in detail.

2.2.1 Existential threat

The perception of an existential threat is what drives a securitization attempt. In line with the inherent requirement of being a lot more specific than any of the usual threats or issues in politics, it "has to be a threat of a dramatic nature, portrayable as threatening the breakdown or ruin of some principle or some other irreparable effect" (Buzan et al. 1998: 27). Objects that are viewed as threatening in general or are unfamiliar to the majority of the public facilitate this depiction. This can be the case with tanks, foreign cultures, minority religions or polluted resources, for example (cf. Buzan et al. 1998: 33). Although highly subjective, this perceived danger is taken seriously by the actor and frequently framed with the argument that "if we do not tackle this problem, everything else will be irrelevant (because we will not be here or will not be free to deal with it in our own way)" (Buzan et al. 1998: 27), thereby dramatising the situation to the extent that the proposed extraordinary measures appear to represent the only possible solution. Consequently, the full attention of a society and all its resources are focused on the containment of this danger, sometimes even in violation of otherwise fundamental rights, such as the right to physical integrity or freedom of expression. The necessary deontic differentiation between 'normal' and 'abnormal' threats and measures can pose a challenge to politicians and other members of society.

However, these extraordinary measures are only admissible in emergency situations when the survival of basic principles and collective units is threatened. In the case of securitization, the principle of 'the more the better' is not applicable as the need for this specific process reflects a prior lack of preparation. Therefore, it seems more like a sign of failure, highlighting the incapacity of routine procedures and institutions (cf. Buzan et al. 1998: 29). On the other hand, securitization and its emergency measures can also become institutionalised. For example, in cases where an existential threat not only poses a sudden, unforeseen danger but is ongoing, securitization becomes institutionalised. In these cases, the audience has accepted that a specific persistent or recurrent issue is inherently urgent and dangerous, and perpetually speak in an affirmatory manner about the issue and the accompanying countermeasures, which can involve elements such as a constantly high security budget or the absence of fundamental rights (cf. Buzan et al. 1998: 27f.). This individual evolution, just like each individual securitization attempt, is highly dependent on meta-variables such as context, culturality and historicity in the society in question. Additionally, the mediality surrounding the securitizing move, especially the framing of the narrative on television and social media, is essential for the audience's acceptance (cf. Pollak et al. 2018: 24ff.). Since the perspective of securitization is only one possible interpretation of a given situation, its threat narrative must factor in all of these contextual elements and the specific society's idiosyncrasies in order to present itself as plausible and compatible with the society's overarching beliefs or experiences. One classic example is the differentiation between foreign troops crossing a border as a peacekeeping force or as hostile troops invading the country (cf. Buzan et al. 1998: 30).

2.2.2 Securitizing actor

To be able to create a convincing narrative and succeed in presenting an issue as "so important that it should not be exposed to the normal haggling of politics but should be dealt with decisively by top leaders prior to other issues" (Buzan et al 1998: 29), a persuasive speaker is necessary. The authors of the securitization framework defined this person as the securitizing agent or securitizing actor. It is somebody who attempts to execute a successful securitizing move by performing a security speech act (cf. Buzan et al 1998: 27). This actor may be an individual or an institution represented by an individual, such as a head of state. While this person typically does not compose their own speeches, they generally provide the strategic direction and key messages, thereby exerting significant influence over the content and framing of securitizing acts. In order to have a realistic chance of success, however, it is necessary for them to exhibit several other qualities. The actor is typically an individual with the authority and platform to speak for a broader collective, e.g. a member of government, a political or religious leader, the head of an international organisation or the media (cf. Sjöstedt 2020: 30). Regardless of gender, age or profession, they need to be influential and trusted leaders for the in-group. In certain cases, the securitizing actor is readily apparent, for instance, when a president delivers a securitizing interview or speech in which they explicitly articulate their role as head of state. However, in other instances, it can be challenging to ascertain whether an individual is speaking on behalf of a government, a department, as a representative of a subgroup or as an individual. Furthermore, it is equally challenging to identify a specific actor in cases where several public figures promote the same or a similar narrative in a combined securitization attempt. One approach is to identify the logic behind the argument and whether it is grounded in an individual or organisational perspective. Another method is to analyse the specific audience and the threatened referent object, which will invariably differ with each threat. A commonality of all actors is their power within the society or system, as it allows them to speak on behalf of a group, movement or for an entire nation (cf. Buzan et al. 1998: 40f.). The authority of these actors derives from their position, resources and perceived legitimacy. It enables them to define what constitutes a threat and to subsequently propose extraordinary measures as a necessary response. This authority plays a crucial role in the process as it grants the credibility and weight required to convince the audience of the speaker's narrative. A head of state or a government official, for example, inherently carry institutional authority, which amplifies the impact of their statements. It also allows them the agency to define strategies or specific countermeasures because of their position. Similarly, the effectiveness of securitization by organisational actors, such as religious leaders, international institutions or influential NGOs, is contingent not only on the actor's words but also on their ability to mobilise the addressees and align their message with the societal values and expectations of their audience.

A **classic example of a securitization constellation** is the nation as the referent object, with the government acting as the securitizing actor. The audience, typically all citizens, has a historical precedent of relying on their representatives and other officials for guidance in the interpretation of current events and potential threats. If the government asserts that an issue poses an existential threat to their survival, citizens are likely to accept this assessment due to the government's access to comprehensive information and experts (cf. Balzacq 2005: 190f.). This intersubjective relationship – along with the trust-instilling institutional context – enhances the authority of the actors, thereby empowering them to establish the narrative of a threatening situation. With their privileged access to the media, these actors are able to disseminate their narrative and further strengthen it dynamically (cf. Rychnovská 2014: 19). Such a large amount of power also brings with it considerable responsibility, which carries ethical implications. Balzacq (2015) argues that the securitization process divides the responsibility between actor and audience in a kind of shared agency because neither works without the other (cf. Balzacq 2005: 190f.). Nevertheless, the most important part of securitization – the decision on its success or failure – falls to the audience.[5] A securitization attempt is successful when the prior, mutually accepted set of rules for behaviour is replaced by new emergency measures that appear more suitable to counter the identified threat, and these are accepted or even actively supported by the target group. For this to occur, the **audience** – in many cases the public – must explicitly agree with the proposed understanding of the situation and the interpretation of the existential threat, which then leads to the implementation of the suggested measures. However, such a degree of acceptance can be difficult to achieve in a democratic system. In particular, the inherent time constraints of most securitization situations prohibit the time-consuming process of reaching a consensus. Concurrently, the measurement of acceptance is challenging. Polls are one method of gauging the percentage of societal support, but they are logistically challenging to administer in times of a perceived immediate

5 On the role of the audience, see also Côté (2016).

need for action. At least, they can document acceptance rates retrospectively, e.g. polls by the Office for National Statistics in the United Kingdom (cf. Vizard 2020; Shepherd et al. 2023). The media can be regarded as another option for determining the acceptance rate within the nation as it is often regarded as a mirror of society (cf. McQuail 2005: 83; Patterson 2008; Ekron 2011: 80; Manzoor 2017: 128). Albeit easily accessible, the accuracy of this approach has not yet been determined in a securitization context. Often, this method is employed in addition to another, more institutionalised way of measuring support, namely political debates and votes. The elected representatives, as proxies for their constituents, are presented with the securitizing actor's threat narrative in the nation's parliament. In these instances, where the head of government delivers a speech to persuade the members of parliament of his perspective, the primary audience comprises the parliament itself, with the general public constituting the secondary audience. Based on this prompt, the elected representatives determine whether to introduce emergency legislation. While this process does not give precise data on the extent of public support, it at least provides a formalised indication of the narrative's resonance within the body of representatives, which traditionally reflects broader societal tendencies and opinions.

In democratic systems, the parliament serves as the formal gatekeeper of securitization, ensuring that extraordinary actions undergo scrutiny and adhere to constitutional principles. While the securitizing move is ostensibly directed at the general public in order to gain widespread acceptance, the crucial institutional mechanism is the parliamentary vote. This duality highlights the complex relationship between public opinion and institutional authority in democratic securitization processes. The general public, as the ultimate audience, provides the societal legitimacy necessary for the actor's narrative to gain traction, while the parliament translates this legitimacy into actionable policy, bridging the gap between mass consent and formal decision-making. The authors of the securitization framework argue that actors strongly associated with their roles can be seen as speakers for the collective they represent rather than as individuals. A president giving a securitizing speech is therefore regarded as speaking for the entire country, rather than speaking as an individual (cf. Buzan et al. 1998: 41). However, the alignment between parliamentary decisions and public opinion may vary depending on factors such as the transparency of the securitization process, the complexity of information, the level of media coverage and the influence of lobbying or party politics. Citizens still possess a variety of avenues through which they can express their opposition to the securitization narrative and the proposed measures, including but not limited to demonstrations, letters and petitions. These actions may potentially result in the reversal of the emergency legislature at a later point in time. Initially, however, the representatives decide on the nation's acceptance of the securitizing actor's narrative of threat. However, it should be noted that this may not be the case for other securitizing actors, such as religious leaders or non-governmental agents. They activate the public through other channels, potentially building a substantial support base. However, the necessary procedure in parliamentary democracies for the enactment of official emergency legislation is usually its passage through parliament, which involves the elected body as primary audience.

Frequently, scholars assume a **homogeneous audience** but this assumption is not verifiable in real cases of securitization (cf. Côté 2016: 450ff.). The supposition that all audience members share the exact same definitive identity disregards the fluid and constructivist nature of identity itself (cf. Peoples and Vaughan-Williams 2021: 18ff.). A securitizing actor framing a perceived threat with this unrealistic assumption is effectively excluding significant segments of the population, e.g. frequently marginalised communities such as disabled citizens or migrants. Consequently, when assessing success, it is imperative to consider the levels of acceptance among the target audience and to identify those groups within the population who have had the capacity to voice significant and realistic objections to the proposed measures. Securitization thus illustrates the power dynamics and distribution of agency within a society. "Rather than thinking of securitization as a mechanism for mobilizing (some fixed and determinate) identity, it may instead be better understood as a mechanism which elicits and encourages identification with particular ideas, notions, or things being subjected to securitization[sic]" (Butler and Wolf 2020: 16).

To sum up, a securitizing move is the communicative action by an actor with considerable authority and power within a given society that presents an object as existentially threatened. The issue only becomes securitized, however, when the audience decides to accept it as such. As public support may prove difficult to measure in a crisis situation, the political securitizing actor operating within a democratic framework must rely on parliamentary approval to substantiate their proposed emergency measures. A successful securitization therefore depends on the willingness of the audience to accept the actor's narrative of an existential threat to a shared value. The attempt becomes successful when the proposed emergency measures are accepted.

2.2.3 Referent object

This willingness on the part of the public is strongly influenced by the selection of the referent object. Traditionally, the object under threat was understood to be the state, closely linked to its territory, government and society, as military survival was the main objective. Securitizing actors can still campaign for the survival of their unit, with the nation state in mind, but can also refer to collective institutions, processes, international structures or organisations, as these affect the internal and external stability of the said state (cf. Buzan et al. 1998: 147). The Copenhagen School, in particular Barry Buzan, Ole Wæver and Jaap de Wilde, expanded this scope to include a broader array of possible objects. These were categorised into five different sectors, as discussed in section 2.2. The authors of the securitization framework remark that they have identified "no necessity for levels to privilege states – the unit level can encompass much more than states" (Buzan et al. 1998: 7). Due to the intersubjective and inherently constructed nature of securitization, the referent object needs to be a commonly valued item that is generally seen as essential for a society. This pre-established respect for the object facilitates the legitimacy of the securitizing actor when they refer to it as threatened. The in-group consensus about the preciousness and importance of the object needs to evolve as part of a discursive process with the society, usually prior to the crisis (cf. Buzan et al. 1998: 31). In principle, anything and anybody can become the referent object of securitization, provided that they fulfil the three criteria of being perceived as a pillar by the audience, of exhibiting a certain degree of stability and of possessing the ability to experience a significant breakdown. By contrast to a merely gradual or barely perceptible disintegration, the threat of a dramatic and substantial collapse of a central principle or another irreparable value can then evoke massive countering reactions (cf. Buzan et al. 1998: 148). The framework's intentional "theoretical plasticity (or vagueness) with regard to what can be the object of security" (Sjöstedt 2019: 30) points to an undefined number of potential applications of securitization theory that are as yet undetermined, as evidenced by the extensive number of studies that have been conducted on the framework, with referent objects ranging from minority rights and migration to health, energy resources or natural disasters (cf. Nyman 2012: 52; Abrahamsen 2005; Hayes 2011; Pour-Ahmadi and Mohseni 2012; Baysa-Barredo 2020; Hapal 2021). In the majority of cases, the referent object is neither situated at a micro level, which would refer to a very small subgroup of citizens, nor at a macro level, which would refer to abstract issues at a state level. Rather, it is located in the middle, between these two extremes (cf. Buzan et al. 1998: 35f.). The question of who or what can be a referent object is a subject of considerable debate among security studies scholars. While it may appear to be a purely theoretical dispute, the selection of the specific object is pivotal in determining how the primary threats to it are understood and which management strategies can be employed. Furthermore, the distinction between the central object being the state or society itself, the individuals within it, or the political system also impacts the definition of security for this entity (cf. Butler and Wolf 2020: 12f.). Whereas actors within the political sector are likely to have the capacity to identify specific spokespeople easily due to their status as elected officials or their position within institutions, other sectors encounter greater difficulty in determining a corresponding securitizing actor. In the majority of cases, more than one securitizing actor claims to be the voice of the threatened audience, which can result in competing threat narratives (cf. Buzan et al 1998: 45).

2.2.4 Speech acts

Securitization can be defined as a discursive process, whereby an issue is transformed into a security matter through the use of linguistic articulation. Buzan, Wæver and de Wilde conceptualise **language** as the essence of securitization, emphasising its role in constructing threats and implementing various stages of security policies. Building on this foundational understanding, they argue that the study of securitization is intrinsically linked to the study of discourse (cf. Buzan et al. 1998: 25). This perspective aligns closely with Austin's speech act theory (cf. section 2.1), which underscores the performative nature of language. Following this framework, the authors contend that securitizing statements function as performative rather than constative utterances, actively shaping the reality they describe (cf. Buzan 2011: 1). Defining the "process of securitization (...) [as] a speech act" (Buzan et al. 1998: 26), they assert that the utterances within a securitizing move do not merely describe or warn about a grave danger but constitute the securitization itself. By labelling an issue as a security and existential threat, the speaker performs the removal of an issue from conventional political proceedings, instead situating it within the context of an emergency characterised by alarmism. In this context, it is implied that political action can no longer be guided by rational or time-consuming deliberation processes but must be quick and decisive. Thus, by labelling an issue as a security concern, an agent claims both a need for and a right to deal with it using extraordinary means (cf. Nyman 2012: 53). Additionally, the rhetorical structure of these securitizing speech acts is characterised by "a specific rhetorical structure stressing urgency, survival and 'priority of action'" (Nyman 2012: 53). Nevertheless, they are not necessarily defined by the use of the term 'security' itself. Instead, the designation of an issue as pressing and an extraordinary existential threat is essential, irrespective of the particular terminology utilised, which may depend on the speaker's rhetorical preferences as well as on the issue itself. This step is crucial not only for persuading the audience but also for justifying certain policies or unfamiliar processes, thus legitimising the subsequent procedural changes that override conventional constraints (cf. Buzan et al. 1998: 27f.).

Although securitization can hardly be measured objectively because security is a discursive construct, there are several **facilitating conditions** for the success of such a speech act. As mentioned above, there are three key conditions – one internal and two external – for a successful speech act in a securitization context. These depend on the addressed group as a successful speech act is necessarily a combination of language and the society in which it is uttered. The first, closely linked to Bourdieu's concept of "cultural capital" (Bourdieu 1991: 107), postulates that the actor must possess sufficient social capital, i.e. authority within the in-group. While this may be due to them holding a specific influential position or being elected, it does not have to be an official position of authority. Rather, this dynamic is contingent on the effective trust and power that the securitizing actor has within the audience. It enables them to convince the audience that their perspective is the correct one. The second external condition refers to the selection of threats that are generally viewed as being threatening by the respective audience, which is necessary for the successful facilitation of securitization. This element can potentially be influenced by the historical and cultural factors inherent within the particular societal context. Lastly, the speaker must adhere to the grammar of security, which consists of a narrative that includes both an existential threat reaching a tipping point where grave consequences for the in-group are impending and a possible solution or at least approaches for mitigating this crisis (cf. Buzan et al. 1998: 32f.). The authors of the securitization framework therefore suggest that the absence of any of these three elements is likely to result in an unsuccessful securitization attempt. However, the inverse is not guaranteed. They concur with Butler (cf. 1996: 40) that the audience's reaction is not always predictable, given that their acceptance of securitization attempts does not follow a fixed plan. Speech acts that have previously been successful, can still fail, even when supported by formal authority, while new actors may unexpectedly succeed in performing securitizing speech acts. Consequently, questions concerning the entities capable of securitization and the determination of securitization occurrences can only be definitively answered retrospectively (cf. Buzan et al. 1998: 46f., see also Vuori 2025).

2.2.5 Criticism and problems

While securitization has been widely recognised as a significant contribution to the study of security and discourse, it has also sparked considerable debate within the academic community. There are three main aspects that have been the subject of criticism. Firstly, there is the Western-centric focus, followed by the emphasis on elite securitizing actors and, finally, the theory's reliance on speech acts.

The first major point of criticism is its **overly Western-centric** perspective. Several basic assumptions, including concepts such as state sovereignty and formalised public debate, are rooted in European or Western political and social structures (cf. Buzan et al. 1998: 30; Wæver et al. 1993: 61ff.). Hence, their applicability across different geopolitical regions has been questioned (cf. Wilkinson 2007: 6f.; Bilgin 2011: 401; Biswas 2013: 89f.). In particular, the theory's "democratic bias" (Vuori 2008: 66) has been challenged on the basis of its assumption of a public sphere where securitization moves are debated and contested. In many non-Western contexts, governance structures, informal power dynamics and cultural norms do not align with this model, thereby rendering its universal application questionable. A corpus-based review by Baele and Jalea (2023) demonstrated that indeed about 75% of scholars working with securitization theory are affiliated with European institutions, predominantly those based in the UK (cf. Baele and Jalea 2023: 385). Its Western-centric bias thus not only limits the framework's explanatory power but also risks the reproduction of hegemonic narratives by marginalising non-Western security discourses and practices. Howell and Richter-Montpetit (2020) even pose the question whether securitization theory could be **considered racist** on the grounds of its perceived inherent civilizationism, antiblack thought and "methodological whiteness" (Howell and Richter-Montpetit 2020: 16). In particular, they claim that in the original framework, Europe is presented as naturally capable of desecuritization in a civilised manner, in contrast to" 'brown' (...) and 'black' (...) regions" (Howell and Richter-Montpetit 2020: 10) of the world, and especially in contrast to a number of weak or failed states where "securitization runs amok" (ibid.). In their **reply**, Wæver and Buzan

(2020; see also Hansen 2020) refute these allegations as misconstructed and mis-attributed (cf. Wæver and Buzan 2020: 388) and call their methodology "deepfake" (Wæver and Buzan 2020: 389) in the sense of picking and choosing quotations without following the intended line of argumentation. In particular, they counter the claim that the presented cases of desecuritization were exclusively from the Global South by mentioning several examples from Northern American and Europe outlined in their respective original framework, some of which explicitly address implications of colonial and postcolonial history (cf. Wæver and Buzan 2020: 389f.). In light of this debate, Innes (2024) proposes to reconceptualise the theory as a tool to focus on power structures, with the intention to explore marginalised groups' experiences of violence that are "made or exposed in the process of securitization" (Innes 2024: 2). However, other scholars such as Sjöstedt (2020) argue that the theory's apparent Eurocentrism may not be inherent in the theory's foundation but rather be scholars' preference due to prevalent academic practice, which needs to expand its focus. She suggests that because of its inherent reflexivity, this framework is actually better suited to cross-cultural utilisation and a broad range of settings than other theories in this context (cf. Sjöstedt 2020: 36). Indeed, the authors of the framework have already included numerous regional actors in their deliberations, among them ASEAN, the South Pacific Forum and the Southern African Development Community (cf. Buzan et al. 1998: 9), in order to demonstrate the efficacy of securitization in such cases. One example of a successful use within a non-democratic setting is Vuori's analysis of the Chinese Tiananmen Square Incident (cf. Vuori 2008: 93f.), others cover African (cf. Osah et al. 2020; Okoli and Ngwu 2022), Arabic (cf. Guéraiche 2022), Middle Eastern (cf. Christou and Aramides 2013; Hoffman 2020; Kikkawa 2024) or Asian (cf. Wang 2021; Omelicheva and Markowitz 2022; Stivas and Sliwinski 2023; Adachi 2024) cases of (de-) securitization.

The second major criticism of securitization is of the theory's narrow focus on **elite actors**. In the words of Wæver et al. (1993), as "'[s]ociety' never speaks, it is only there to be spoken for" (Wæver et al. 1993: 188), which means that the identification of issues and the communication of the public's needs and desires becomes the task of politicians. Consequently, securitization prioritises the speech acts and discourse of elite actors, such as elected politicians and state officials, by stressing their authority and agency in decision-making while neglecting the role of the audience itself and of voices from non-elite and civil society actors when it comes to shaping security discourses. Their possible contributions, dissent or protest are not part of the securitization framework. This perspective has been criticised by Thierry Balzacq (2019), among others, who argues that the attribution of roles in this theory resembles the distribution of power between sovereign and subjects more closely than that between speaker and audience. He does not identify the decision on the success or failure of a securitization attempt as being one made by the audience but rather agrees with Huysmans (cf. 2011: 375) that the postulated balance of power rather appears to be tilted in favour of the securitizing actor. This effectively positions the audience as passive spectators rather than active contributors to the policy-making process (cf. Balzacq 2019: 341f.). However, Côté's meta-study of articles on securitization (2016) found evidence for both passive and active audiences, the latter having successfully brought about modifications to the securitizing move through iterative interactions (cf. Côté 2016: 546; Sjöstedt 2020: 37).

Additionally, other scholars, such as Charrett (cf. 2009: 29) and Rosoux (cf. 2019: 203), have expressed discontent with the theory's constricted perspective on potential speakers, while still acknowledging the framework's value for security studies. "Once (...) dislodged from its narrow focus on state elites it can actively fulfil its potential to locate securitizing actors at the sub- and supra- state level[sic]" (Charrett 2009: 26). They argue for a broader approach encompassing discourse contributions from minority groups and civil actors not holding official positions, such as victim's associations. Often, these are not recognised due to their lesser authority and limited resources, demonstrating the power relations that exist within the respective society or group. Consequently, these authors propose that those marginalised or alternative actors who may articulate different speech acts compared to prominent, more vocal officials – or who may even engage in counter-securitization or resistance – need to be proactively sought out when examining a securitization discourse and determining its success (cf. Charrett 2009: 29).

Building on this, the third key criticism concerns securitization's extensive **reliance on speech act theory.** The authors' underlying assertion that "the way to study securitization is to study discourse" (Buzan et al. 1998: 25) is regarded as reductive, as it fails to take into account non-discursive practices. Stritzel argues that "the performative power of a speech act cannot be captured only in the abstract and in the form of a single linguistic act, but needs to be contextually located within broader structures" (Stritzel 2014: 46). He therefore proposes an expansion of the analytical scope to encompass non-linguistic practices and material factors. In agreement with Stritzel, Balzacq (2011) emphasises the necessity of considering the dynamic between discursive and non-discursive elements, such as visual representations and material actions, which may frequently play a substantial role in securitization processes. For instance, the non-verbal deployment of military forces, the erection of physical barriers or the implementation of surveillance technologies can communicate and reinforce a securitizing move just as effectively as a speech act (cf. Balzacq 2011: 8; see also Engelkamp et al. 2020). Additionally, Sjöstedt et al. (2019) point out that even officials in leading positions may not always be able to articulate their concerns and opinions freely, possibly being subject to discrimination on the basis of race or gender, or fearing repercussions by political opponents, their own party or group, or violent groups in society (cf. Sjöstedt et al. 2019: 571). Moreover, the significance of cultural meaning should not be overlooked in favour of textual meaning. The actor's speech acts need to be interpreted within the context of the target audience's historically accumulated knowledge and cultural practices (cf. Balzacq 2011: 4). By focusing primarily on language, the theory risks neglecting these material and performative dimensions, which are integral to the construction and maintenance of security narratives. Consequently, scholars have advocated for a more comprehensive approach that combines both linguistic and extralinguistic practices to provide a fuller understanding of securitization dynamics (cf. McDonald 2008: 568).

3 Intersection Between Speech Acts and Securitization in Political Discourse

Securitization is an established part of any society's political discourse. In contrast, even though speech act theory is well established in pragmatics and researched from a variety of perspectives, it is still rare in the study of political discourse (cf. Marsen and Ali-Chand 2022: 25; see also chapter 4). However, Arsith (2015) argues that political discourse utilises and exploits the characteristics of speech acts exceptionally well (cf. Arsith 2015: 622).

First, their contextual determination, in particular the cultural and spatio-temporal conditions, together with the characteristics of an utterance's audience significantly influence its reception. A similar phenomenon can be observed in political discourse, resulting in diverse presentations and outcomes regarding the same issue in different cultures or societies. Invariably, the speaker's message needs to be interpreted by the audience, which may lead to individual listeners coming to a different understanding, depending on their position, status, socio-cultural background, demographic and individual factors, or knowledge of a given topic. Additionally, the conventionality of speech acts demands several felicity conditions, which can also be transferred to political discourse (cf. Arsith 2015: 621). In addition to the recipient, the elements of the speaker's status and intention as well as the circumstances of the utterance determine whether the desired effect can be achieved. Analogous mechanisms can be observed in political discourse, where the efficacy of agenda setting is found to be contingent upon the degree of influence a societal actor holds. Meanwhile, speech acts possess the inherent capacity to transform the nature of something. This dimension is of particular significance within the context of political discourse as it has the potential to motivate citizens to actively engage with the objective of changing the world. Therefore, all these components of illocutionary force are also activated in political discourse (cf. Arsith 2015: 622). It is thus surprising that speech act theory is rarely applied to research within the area of political discourse.

This study aims to narrow this gap. It focuses on speech acts in a small, specific area of political discourse: securitization. Buzan, Wæver and de Wilde explicitly link their securitization framework to Austin's speech act theory and emphasise the performativity of securitizing speech acts, wherein language not only describes a reality but actively creates it (cf. Buzan et al. 1998: 32). A securitizing actor declares an issue to be an existential threat through a speech act, thereby attempting to shift it from the realm of normal politics into the realm of emergency measures. This performativity aligns closely with Austin's and Searle's notion of illocutionary acts, where the act of saying something is simultaneously the act of doing something. Thus, the illocution constitutes the core of the securitizing move by presenting something as threatened, whereas the perlocution focuses on the effect of the speech acts afterwards, i.e. the measures the acts entail (cf. Balzaq 2015: 109).

Securitization is a process that can be accompanied by a variety of speech acts. The attempt to persuade the target audience of the narrative of threat begins with the securitizing actor conveying a sense of fear and urgency, emphasising the gravity of a perceived threat. They proceed to explain the danger and its implications for the in-group. The audience is urged to adopt specific behaviours that deviate from established norms or practices in order to address the crisis, while the speaker highlights their personal commitment to specific actions (cf. Buzan et al. 1998: 26). Ultimately, if the audience is persuaded, the actor may formally declare a state of emergency or implement countermeasures. It is evident that this process's success relies on the audience's compliance and acceptance.

However, the application of speech act theory within the securitization framework goes beyond individual utterances to encompass the broader discursive practices that support the construction of security threats. The "grammar of security" described by Buzan, Wæver and de Wilde (1998: 33) requires the speaker to construct a narrative that resonates with the audience's cultural and social context, aligning the speech act with both internal linguistic rules and external socio-political conditions. Furthermore, the intersubjective nature of securitization (cf. Balzacq 2015: 108), with success depending on the audience's acceptance, highlights the role of context and reception. These aspects are also central to the pragmatic study of speech acts, again demonstrating the close relationship between the two theories.

However, only a limited number of studies integrate speech act theory into the analysis of securitization, combining linguistic and security studies in an interdisciplinary approach. Among the most notable contributions are the works of Marsen and Ali-Chand (2022) as well as Schueler and Marx's (2023), both of which examine speech acts in political discourse during the COVID-19 pandemic.

In their research, Marsen and Ali-Chand (2022) analyse political speech acts in crisis communication by comparing the discursive strategies employed by the heads of government in Australia, Fiji and New Zealand in selected speeches. Despite the absence of any reference to securitization theory, they focus on speeches delivered over a three-month period during the initial phase of the pandemic. Utilising Searle's speech act typology, they identify directives as the most commonly used speech act, followed by declaratives, assertives and warnings. Nevertheless, the temporal constraints inherent in the study's design prevent a deeper investigation into long-term patterns in securitizing discourse.

In contrast, Schueler and Marx (2023) conduct an in-depth analysis of all Dutch COVID-19 press conferences, spanning the 13 months from March 2020 to April 2021. Their study examines speech acts performed by 11 government officials, including Prime Minister Rutte and Minister of Health, Welfare and Sport de Jonge, alongside their interactions with over 150 journalists. The authors findings indicate that assertives dominate the discourse, with directives (both modest and strong) ranking second, followed by commissives, expressives and declaratives being least frequent. A notable observation is that the prime minister utilises more expressives, directives and declaratives in comparison to the health minister, who relies more on commissives and assertives. Furthermore, the study identifies structural patterns within the press conferences, showing parallels between briefings that lift restrictions and those that impose them. However, the incorporation of almost 170 speakers in the dataset makes it difficult to draw clear conclusions about the actual securitizing statements made by the Prime Minister and the Minister of Health. Moreover, the inherent nature of the dialogue represented in this corpus is not representative of typical communicative processes in securitization attempts.

Other studies provide only isolated observations of speech acts during the securitizing move. One example is **Majeed's (2022)** research. She examines speech acts in a speech by US President Trump in March 2020. Although this statement is taken from the securitizing period for this country, the informative value of the analysis is limited by its focus on a single speech.

Consequently, it offers a selective portrayal of the president's early securitizing communication during the pandemic, precluding the analysis of characteristics that manifest over a more extended period.

Studies such as that of AlAfnan and Oshchepkova (2022) examine speech acts in the context of other securitizing actors. Their analysis focuses on the UN Secretary-General as a securitizing agent, specifically assessing his opening remarks at the Emergency Special Session on Ukraine (cf. AlAfnan and Oshchepkova 2022: 96). However, this approach differs from other studies in terms of its intended audience, as it is not directed at citizens of a nation but rather at representatives at the UN General Assembly. As with Majeed (2022), the reliance on a single speech limits the insights that can be drawn regarding Guterres's securitizing discourse. As a result, this dataset does not allow for the identification of broader patterns of securitization, making generalisation unfeasible.

4 Research Design

4.1 Gap in research

It can be observed that the existing literature on securitization has largely neglected the pragmatic dimension of the securitization process. Although the authors of the original securitization framework already acknowledged the role of speech acts in this process, explicitly referencing Austin's speech act theory (cf. Buzan et al. 1998: 26), this aspect has been largely sidelined in security studies and political science. Concurrently, the securitization aspect itself has been largely overlooked in linguistic research. To date, there has been no study that provides a systematic empirical analysis of the specific speech acts used in successful securitization. Furthermore, a **significant gap** remains in the literature regarding characteristic speech act patterns in the securitizing move or the prototypical speech act structure of a securitizing statement. This lack of research prevents a comprehensive understanding of the manner in which securitizing utterances contribute to the linguistic construction of security threats. Consequently, a systematic, empirically grounded investigation into the speech acts in successful securitization is essential to illuminate the linguistic processes involved in the initial stages of securitization, contributing to a more nuanced understanding of the process from a linguistic perspective.

4.2 Research questions

This dissertation project aims to close the gap in existing research with an empirical research of speech acts in the securitizing move to describe the process from a linguistic point of view. The following two research questions will therefore be investigated:

1. Which speech acts are used by a securitizing actor during a securitizing move?
2. What is the prototypical structure of speech acts in the securitizing speeches delivered by British Prime Minister Boris Johnson during the COVID-19 pandemic?

In order to respond to these two questions, a case study of securitizing speech acts will be conducted, employing methods rooted in corpus-assisted discourse analysis. The object of this analysis is the official communication of British Prime Minister Boris Johnson during the initial phase of the COVID-19 pandemic.

Since different crisis settings may impact the choice of speech acts utilised by the securitizing actor, this thesis focuses on a single case of securitization. The **COVID-19 pandemic** has been selected as a recent and particularly pervasive example of successful national securitization. As a result of its perceived threat to public health and the NHS, the SARS-CoV-2 virus was securitized by the government, prompting the implementation of extensive emergency measures affecting all citizens (cf. section 5.1). Furthermore, this specific instance of securitization is particularly conducive to further research. Given its global nature, the insights derived from this British example can be readily extended to other case studies, facilitating future comparison with findings from other varieties of English or different languages and cultures.

In general, securitization is a task that only influential actors "in a position of authority" (Buzan et al. 1998: 33) can hope to succeed in. At a national, let alone at the international level, typically only "political leaders, bureaucracies, [or] governments" (ibid.: 40) assume the role of securitizing actors. As head of state, the **British prime minister** exercises the highest authority and speaks directly on behalf of the government. Consequently, Johnson's speeches are likely to encapsulate the government's key arguments and exhibit greater focus than parliamentary debates, social media content or speeches by local officials, who may represent diverse interests and perspectives. Moreover, McClaughlin et al. (2021) show that Johnson was the leading figure in the governmental securitization of COVID-19 in the UK, with all other ministers delivering significantly fewer speeches (cf. McClaughlin et al. 2021: 2). Furthermore, prime ministerial speeches typically attract greater media attention, which results in a more effective dissemination of the content among the general public. Bearing in mind that the public's focus was primarily on their nation's leading politicians during the pandemic, in continuation of what McAllister called the "personalization of politics" (2007: 572), these factors reinforce the impact of securitization. Therefore, this analysis will limit its scope to an examination of the prime minister's speech acts in his official press statements during the pandemic.

This study is exclusively concerned with the initial phase of securitization, the securitizing move. The underlying rationale is that the success of a securitization attempt depends on the ability of the securitizing actor to present the threat in a way that is perceived as being damaging enough to justify the proposed countermeasures. If this is not achieved, the audience is unlikely to accept the proposed measures, leading to the failure of the attempt (cf. section 2.2). It is thus evident that this initial phase, and particularly its speech acts, are of paramount importance as they determine whether the securitization will be successful and proceed to the subsequent stages. Therefore, this analysis focuses on Johnson's speech acts in this first phase of the pandemic.

The **first research question** aims to identify the specific speech acts that are utilised in the initial stage of securitization. A case study of a successful securitization is employed to identify them. They are analysed according to Searle's pre-established speech act categories (cf. section 2.1.6). The **second research question** aims to identify the characteristic speech act patterns that were employed in the exemplary case study. Identifying the linguistic mechanisms that systematically present the threat as an urgent security issue and persuade the public to implement exceptional measures will provide insights into how public compliance was achieved and sustained over time. In this context, 'characteristic' is used to refer to the most frequent individual speech acts and the most common categories to be able to state which sets of speech acts are typical of a securitizing move by the prime minister in a situation such as the COVID-19 pandemic.

By answering these two research questions, this research seeks to highlight not only the linguistic strategies employed to establish and maintain the security narrative but also to illuminate the broader impact of such discourse on public resilience and governmental authority. This approach will facilitate a more nuanced understanding of the manner in which speech acts contribute to the alignment of public perception with governmental objectives, particularly in the context of an ongoing, high-stakes crisis such as a pandemic.

4.3 Methodology

4.3.1 Corpus-Assisted Discourse Analysis

The methodology of **corpus-assisted discourse analysis** (CADA) has been selected. This approach of mixing corpus linguistics (CL) and critical discourse analysis (CDA) has become increasingly popular in the last 20 years and is referred to in the literature by several names. While some researchers, among them Alan Partington, use 'corpus-assisted discourse studies', or CADS for short (cf. Partington 2007; Jaworska 2016), Baker employs the term 'corpus-assisted discourse analysis' (cf. Baker 2020). For this study, the term 'corpus-assisted discourse analysis' (CADA) has been chosen because of its explicit focus on the analytical element. This choice is in line with recent works by Taylor (2014), Griebel and Volkmann (2019), Baker (2020), Matthews (2021), Attia (2022), Yu et al. (2023), Pei and Cheng (2024) as well as Nervino et al. (2025), to name just a few.

The critical discourse analysis (CDA) method, as developed by Wodak, is widely regarded as an effective approach for qualitative data analysis (cf. Weiss and Wodak 2003; Baker et al. 2008; Wodak and Meyer 2016; Ammoussou and Allagbe 2018; Catalano and Waugh 2020). However, as already described in 1995 by Hardt-Mautner, "the mainly qualitative methodology used in CDA proved ill-suited to handling the sizeable corpus that formed the basis of the study" (Hardt-Mautner 1995: 1). It therefore seems beneficial to employ complementary corpus linguistics methods in order to add a more quantitative insight into larger corpora. Charlotte Taylor and Alan Partington, among others, have demonstrated on several occasions that complex studies can benefit from a combination of methods from corpus linguistics and critical discourse analysis (cf. Partington et al. 2013: 12; Taylor 2013; Mautner 2016). As CDA is most suitable for smaller corpora, representativeness is a critical issue in such analyses. It is essential to remain aware that a corpus element has been selected based on specific characteristics to ensure that these are not presented as typical afterwards (cf. Hardt-Mautner 1995: 3; Mautner 2007: 54). "Relying on large amounts of data and computer-aided techniques does not bring objectivity, but it can provide greater accuracy and accountability" (Marchi and Taylor 2018: 7), as the process leading to the interpretation of results is reproducible. Consequently, combining CDA with methods from CL enables the investigation of typicality with statistical evidence, thereby enhancing the reliability of the findings. However, their combined approach should not be simply reduced to a mere fusion of quantitative and qualitative methods and perspectives. Baker et al. (2008) describe CL as a set of techniques that are applied to corpora, i.e. large, electronically-stored collections of real-life texts. Despite the prevalence of statistical software in many standard methods, the precise selection of queries remains a qualitative decision-making process. This involves interpreting examples from concordances and determining the limits of statistical significance (cf. Baker et al. 2008: 273f.). Therefore, the "natural synergy" (Sinclair 2004: 11) of these overlapping approaches enable research interests that encompass both questions about the presence and quantity of specific linguistic elements in a text as well as the subsequent investigation of their raison d'être and circumstances (cf. Baker et al. 2008: 281, see also Flowerdew 2012). Their non-standardised repertoire of available methods and procedures, which are by no means limited to close reading for CDA and frequency analysis for CL, concentrate on identifying and interpreting unusual patterns by using a range of tools within their respective contexts.

Statistical insights into a dataset permit CADA researchers to readily identify keywords or structures of interest, which they can then examine qualitatively (cf. Mautner 2007: 56). This provides a seamless and data-driven entry into the analytical process. Another benefit of integrating the two approaches is their broadened focus. While CDA is generally employed for smaller textual units, CL techniques have now made it possible to analyse larger datasets without compromising the quality of the analysis. CADA allows for the illustration of complex linguistic choices during the production of corpus elements, such as political speeches, facilitated by the computational power and speed of modern software. The previous criticism of CL as being solely descriptive and neglecting contextual relations (cf. Mautner 2007: 55) can be addressed by incorporating CDA elements into the analysis, with the reverse advantage that CL concordance lines root an interpretation into plausible contexts, consequently enabling reproducibility. The distinctive benefit of such a combination of the two approaches is therefore that qualitative findings can be quantified and quantitative results contextualised and interpreted, thus enabling nuanced answers to research questions than would otherwise be impossible.

The **limitations** of this approach have been clearly stated from the beginning, with Hardt-Mautner articulating her concerns as early as 1995. First, the generalisation of findings is closely interwoven with corpus size and data selection. In order to make valid general statements about any language, it is necessary to have access to a corpus of a considerable size, usually comprising millions of words, with the exact number depending on the respective research question. The generation of such corpora is a lengthy, time-consuming and complex process, which is why the majority of researchers employ pre-existing corpora or compile smaller, specialised corpora themselves. However, flaws in the compilation process or biases may result in a lack of representativeness. "The smaller the corpus, the more modest the claims must be" (Hardt-Mautner 1995: 23), even though with specialised corpora, this reduced size might nonetheless signify a salient analysis of a certain genre or variety. Hardt-Mautner's initial concern about working with untagged corpora and only counting specific phenomena that are easily detectable with basic software tools (cf. Hardt-Mautner 1995: 23) has since been alleviated, given the availability of refined modern software, such as *AntConc* or *R*, and automated annotation software, such as *SketchEngine* or *TagAnt*, most of which are available free of charge online. Nevertheless, the deployment of these instruments necessitates a certain degree of expertise and, in some cases, a set of specially prepared data. In certain instances, researchers continue to annotate their dataset themselves as the existing tag sets do not seem sophisticated enough or the desired level of annotation is not yet automated.

4.3.2 Corpora in research

A robust CADA analysis is contingent upon the utilisation of a **carefully designed corpus**. This is defined as "large, principled collection[s] of naturally-occurring texts that [are](...) stored in electronic form (accessible on computer). Corpora can include both written and transcribed spoken texts" (Conrad 2002: 76). In general, the objective is to create a corpus that is representative of the particular linguistic area under investigation (cf. Cheng 2012: 67). The criteria for compiling a corpus are thus usually rigorous, detailed and formulated prior to the data-mining process. Ädel (2021) outlines several core principles for this. It is vital that the corpus is compiled in a consistent manner, with all elements of a certain characteristic included or excluded in a transparent and systematic way. This approach must be taken in order to ensure comprehensive coverage of all relevant aspects, thus making the corpus a representative sample of the phenomenon of interest that exhibits a balanced distribution of its components (cf. Ädel 2021: 4ff.; see also Sinclair 2005: 2ff.; Cheng 2012: 4).

The **size of a corpus** is typically measured in words, with the synchronic *Corpus of Contemporary American English* (COCA) currently being the largest general corpus, comprising one billion words structured in eight different genres (cf. Davies 2022). A corpus for the British variety of English from the late twentieth century is the *British National Corpus* (BNC), a synchronic dataset with more than 100 million words (cf. BNC 2022). These are general corpora aiming to represent the full variety of English, comprising millions of words. In contrast, there are also specialised corpora that usually encompass a much smaller sample of a language, e.g. the *Wikipedia Corpus*, which consists of the entire English-language part of the internet encyclopaedia (cf. Davies 2015), or the *Coronavirus Corpus*, an ongoing collection of news articles on COVID-19 (cf. Davies 2019). Commonly employed for a diverse range of research purposes, such as lexicography and language pedagogy, specialised corpora are relatively modest in size, typically ranging from a few thousand to a few million words (cf. Cheng 2012: 32), and are more narrowly focused on a specific research interest, e.g. insights into a certain register, a specific situation or a regional dialect (cf. Weisser 2015: 21).

Corpora can be **annotated,** e.g. for parts of speech, facilitating the identification of grammatical patterns. Additionally, there are pragmatically annotated corpora indicating speech acts or other pragmatically relevant information (cf. ibid: 24; see also Subramanian et al. 2019). The manual annotation process, which has historically been a time-consuming endeavour, can now be carried out automatically through the utilisation of appropriate software in some cases. One example is the use of *SketchEngine* or *TagAnt* for the annotation of parts of speech. However, this requires an extensive pre-modelled tag set, which is often not available for less common pragmatic annotation requests, such as individual speech acts.

4.3.3 Compilation of the research corpus

This analysis is based on a specialised corpus consisting of official communication by the British government during the COVID-19 pandemic. To ensure coherence, the corpus has been compiled with five rigorous **criteria**:

- a single topic,
- a single speaker,
- solely instances of direct speech,
- a single source, and
- a pre-set timeframe.

It thus comprises all press statements on the subject of the pandemic made by the British prime minister that were published on the official government website during the ten-month period under investigation. This special corpus will be referred to as the **Johnson Pandemic Corpus 2020**, abbreviated ***JPanC20,*** in the following.

In this context, the term '**press statement**' denotes official communication issued in the personal words of the prime minister. It has been selected to differentiate from the broader "press release" (Cambridge Dictionary 2024a) by placing emphasis on the active role of the prime minister in disseminating information in accordance with the official governmental wording for these instances (cf. Johnson 2020a: 1). Press statements given at press conferences, which are considered a formalised form of political communication (cf. Jarren and Donges 2011: 243), are frequently used for the analysis of political language or narratives. These statements are characterised by an informative-persuasive intention and typically encompass a range of speech acts, including motivating, thanking or warning the audience (cf. Diehr and Stiglbauer 2021: 45f.).

In the corpus compiled for this research, the **primary addressee** is the general British public. Nevertheless, in accordance with the principle of inclusivity, the content also encompasses addresses presented in the British Parliament to a smaller audience of representatives or delivered in the General Assembly of the United Nations. For the sake of representativeness, these were not excluded as they were published via the official communication channel in the period under investigation. In order to ensure that the intended speech acts are as unfiltered as possible – so that the most authentic representation of the statements is provided – all press releases that either merely summarise the content of a speech or engagement, only cite select parts of a speech or report the words of other government officials have been excluded from the corpus.

At the outset of the COVID-19 pandemic, Boris Johnson was the prime minister of the United Kingdom.[1] The *JPanC20* is made up of his speeches, which form the basis for this investigation. Given that press conferences were the principal mode of top-down communication with the public at that time, the corpus consists of the official published versions of the prime minister's statements, sourced directly from the UK government's official communication platform, https://www.gov.uk/search/news-and-communications. They can be accessed via the 'government activity' section under the header 'News stories, speeches, letters and notices' (cf. Government of the UK 2024). Each document contains a transcript of Johnson's utterances, accompanied by metadata detailing the date and context of each statement, e.g. an oral

1 For detailed insight into his political style, see e.g. Charteris-Black (2019).

statement to parliament or a public address. Moreover, the webpage of each corpus document states that it is a "[t]ranscript of the speech, exactly as it was delivered" (Johnson 2020a: 1; see also all other corpus elements).

Considering Mollin's (2007: 208) concerns regarding the linguistic accuracy of transcripts of political statements created for purposes other than linguistic investigation, the authenticity of the corpus elements has been investigated nonetheless. Given that Boris Johnson delivers prewritten speeches in 38 of the 46 corpus elements, which are supplemented by two newspaper articles that also serve to disseminate the desired content in an intentional manner, it can be presupposed that Johnson's utterances reflect his intended messaging as they are not products of spontaneous speech, as would be the case in parliamentary debates. Additionally, the corpus includes one video of a personal statement by Johnson. Its transcript has been obtained from the official website but has also been verified manually against the original video on X (cf. Johnson [@BorisJohnson] 2020). With the exception of two instances of 'uh' that are absent from the official transcript, the content remains consistent, which aligns with the nature of pre-recorded videos as they can be revised and are only uploaded when deemed satisfactory by the speaker. This process minimises repetitions and mispronunciations that might feature in extemporaneous remarks. Lastly, statements delivered in the House of Commons, where the inherently dialogic exchange may introduce more features of spontaneous spoken language, constitute only five documents within the corpus, a relatively limited portion of the dataset. However, the presence of some repetition in these elements (cf. Johnson 2020t: 3) suggests that such redactions, if applied, were minimal. By contrast, the transcripts in general lack markers for short or longer pauses, usually indicated by commas or full stops, as well as for filled pauses, which are traditionally marked by 'uh' or 'uhm' (cf. Mollin 2007: 193). While these factors may result in a transcript that differs slightly from the actual delivery, this study is not concerned with the characteristics of spoken language but rather with the strategic use and distribution of speech acts within the prime minister's statements. Therefore, the absence of these markers does not affect the analysis. Although they might have undergone minimal editing, it appears that these elements are still effective in capturing the essence of the intended communicative acts and exhibit the performative nature of the speeches as conveyed to the audience. Consequently, the transcripts have been deemed reliable representations of the speech acts that formed the basis of the government's official messaging.

The focus of the analysis is on the securitizing move, which is completed once the securitizing actor's interpretation of the situation has been accepted by a significant proportion of the public and the subsequent stage of executing securitization measures is reached (cf. Buzan et al. 1998: 31). In the case of the COVID-19 pandemic, this applies to the **period** from the first infections, where politicians attempted to persuade citizens of the situation's gravity, until the point at which their measures had been accepted. Thus, the earliest press statement included in the dataset represents the first mention of COVID-19 in a speech of Johnson's, delivered on 3 March 2020. The point at which vaccines became publicly available has been chosen as the endpoint to this stage, as the key message for the first part of the pandemic in the United Kingdom had been to stay strong until vaccines "get our economies moving again, and allow us to reclaim our lives" (Johnson 2020as: 1). The final element in the *JPanC20* is therefore the speech delivered by the prime minister on 2 December 2020, in which he announced the approval of the first vaccine for distribution across the United Kingdom. The first Briton was vaccinated six days later, on 8 December (cf. Murray 2020: 1). Consequently, these criteria result in the formation of a corpus that encompasses the period from mid-March to early December 2020, comprising 46 statements on the COVID-19 virus issued by Prime Minister Johnson, which were published on the official government communications website.

Following the compilation of the corpus, its elements were **edited** for linguistic purposes. This involved the removal of any images and links within the documents, leaving only the header, which includes the date and title, as well as the content of the statement. A copy of this version of the *JPanC20* has been saved in .txt files for the purpose of ensuring compatibility with quantitative tools, such as *AntConc*.

Subsequently, the corpus was **annotated** for speech acts. In accordance with Saldaña's (2013) recommendations, the initial stage of the process entailed an in-depth examination of the entire dataset, with a particular focus on identifying the broad narratives (cf. Saldaña 2013: 58ff.). Using the coding tool within the software *MAXQDA* (cf. Verbi 2024a), each utterance in the 46 statements was then subjected to a first coding cycle. Following Searle's taxonomy of illocutionary acts (cf. section 2.1.6), his five categories were taken as a deductive starting point and subsequently divided into subcategories, enabling a more nuanced examination. While the initial subcategory structure (cf. table A1) was informed by the framework proposed by Marsen and Ali-Chand (cf. 2022: 8), extensive modifications were made on an inductive basis in a first round of coding in order to better reflect the distinctive characteristics and contextual features of the *JPanC20*. In accordance with the established standards of corpus linguistics, a second coding cycle was conducted to guarantee consistency and selectivity across the various subcategories (cf. Saldaña 2013: 58ff.; Stefanowitsch 2020: 122). As a result, a pragmatically annotated corpus is obtained, with each sentence containing none, one or multiple speech acts.

5 Case Study

Beginning with a brief outline of the key characteristics of the pandemic securitization in the case of Great Britain in 2020, the context of the case study is explained. Then, the corpus analysis commences with an introduction to the characteristics of the corpus, providing key data such as the chronological distribution of statements over the course of the observation period. The following application of corpus linguistics methods to the dataset offers preliminary insights into the main themes and narratives. Starting with the **analysis of word frequencies** in section 5.3.1, the tone and recurring clusters within the most frequent 100 words are analysed, providing some first information about the specialised corpus (cf. Baron et al. 2009: 41). The subsequent **keyword analysis** (cf. section 5.3.2) enables an understanding of the context of the most frequent words and may already offer insights into the "patterns of language" (Conrad 2002: 77). The keyness rate is calculated for the individual corpus types in comparison to a reference corpus, identifying words that exhibit a greater difference in relative frequency. As the χ2-measure has been demonstrated to become unreliable in cases where the expected frequency does not reach the threshold of five occurrences, Log-Likelihood (LL) has been determined as the more reliable statistic for this calculation because this threshold cannot be ruled out for this analysis (cf. Pojanapunya and Watson Todd 2016: 146f.). All keyness calculations were conducted automatically using the software *AntConc*, which offers a keyword ranking system based on the LL metric (cf. Anthony 2023: 1).

For this specialised corpus comprising official government statements in British English, the *BE06 Corpus of British English*, produced by Paul Baker of Lancaster University, is designated as the **reference corpus** (cf. Baker 2009). Given the relatively recent publication date, its size and the diverse range of content types represented in this corpus of general British English, this specific reference corpus is deemed an appropriate choice for the reference corpus in this particular study.

Several other corpora were considered. The *Hansard Corpus* represents another potential option, given its comprehensive coverage of parliamentary speeches dating from circa 1800 to 2005. This corpus encompasses approximately 1.6 billion words in total, as documented by Davies (2015). Nevertheless, considering that Prime Minister Johnson's press statements were not confined to the House of Commons but were predominantly delivered outside of that setting and to a different audience, this option was deemed unsuitable. Additionally, the aforementioned limitations identified by Mollin (2007) suggest that the Hansard Corpus may not be a suitable reference corpus for the entire variety of British English.

As another possibility, the *British National Corpus* (BNC), the largest and most comprehensive corpus of British English, was considered. It includes approximately 100 million words and encompasses a diverse range of genres – both spoken and written – including fiction, magazines, newspapers and academic texts. Originally compiled by the Oxford University Press, the corpus encompasses the period from the 1980s to 1993, offering a representative sample of British English. However, the content is more reflective of the language variety of the late twentieth century and may not capture the nuances of contemporary lexicon and syntax. Consequently, the *BE06* corpus was identified as the most appropriate reference corpus for this new specialised corpus comprising press statements made by Boris Johnson in 2020.

In the following, the examination of speech acts is initiated with a description of the distribution of speech act categories. In accordance with the structure of Searle's preliminary five categories, i.e. assertives, expressives, commissives, directives and declaratives, a comprehensive investigation of speech acts is conducted, starting with the most frequent category. The corresponding subcategories within each category are similarly examined in order of frequency and illustrated through examples in order to contextualise them within the corpus in sections 5.4.1 to 5.4.5. This part of the analysis aims to address the first research question, which concerns the types of speech acts employed by the securitizing actor in the securitizing move. The contextualised description of all speech acts present in this case study provides an empirical overview of these illocutionary acts. Building on these results, a meta-analysis is conducted in section 5.4.6 to examine the characteristics of the *JPanC20*. First, the press statements with the greatest and least number of speech acts are contextualised.

The study then introduces a novel metric, the **Speech Act-Token-Ratio** (SATR), which has not been previously described in the literature. This metric has been developed to measure speech act density in a document or corpus by calculating the proportion of speech acts to tokens within the respective unit, enabling a comparison across different corpora or corpus elements. It is generated by dividing the total number of speech acts in one analysed unit by the number of tokens it contains.

Therefore, the SATR is calculated using the following formula:

$$\text{SATR} = \frac{\text{number of speech acts}}{\text{number of tokens}}$$

The resulting value ranges from 1 (where each token constitutes its own speech act) to 0.00...01 (where the entire corpus consists of one single speech act). This value illustrates the speech act density in the element under examination.

The inverse calculation – dividing the number of tokens by the number of speech acts – yields the average length of a speech act in the unit. Together, these metrics offer a nuanced comparative perspective on the distribution and density of speech acts, thereby enhancing the analysis of pragmatic structures in a dataset. Unlike other measures of discourse complexity, such as the type-token ratio (TTR), the SATR specifically highlights communicative variety in terms of pragmatic functions, thereby providing a focused lens on speech act density.

The analysis continues with a description of the most frequent speech acts, both in regard to individual speech acts and to subcategories across all five categories. The objective of this process is to identify the characteristic utterances and patterns that were utilised in the prime minister's successful securitizing move. The study proceeds with the examination of co-occurring speech acts in section 5.4.6.3, once more divided into categories, thus shedding light on the underlying content relations and identifying speeches that are characterised by a high number of overlapping speech acts. Lastly, the distribution of speech act categories is examined over the different segments of the speeches in section 5.4.6.4. This step employs a tripartite structure, focusing on the initial, middle and concluding parts, to investigate the distribution of speech acts across speeches in relation to the specific phase of the pandemic. In this context, particular attention is paid to the precise sequence of speech acts at two pivotal positions: firstly, the initiating utterances in the *JPanC20*, and secondly, the final speech act of each press statement, as these typically reiterate the statement's core message. This second part of the analysis attempts to answer the second research question on characteristic speech acts in this case of securitization. Consequently, it examines whether the securitizing actor follows a particular pattern of speech act categories – or even individual speech acts – in his speeches in order to identify elements that may contribute to the success of the securitization process. The findings are subsequently brought together, summarised and interpreted in chapter 6.

5.1 Securitizing the COVID-19 Pandemic in Great Britain

This study uses the British government's communication of the threat posed by the COVID-19 pandemic as an example of a successful securitization. The reasons for this are outlined below.

The first patients exhibiting symptoms caused by the virus later called 'COVID-19' were confirmed in Great Britain by 28 January 2020 (cf. Aspinall 2021: 1). At that time, the government's focus remained primarily on Brexit negotiations (cf. Johnson 2020au) and initially, the virus was not treated as a pressing concern. Lilleker and Stoekle even diagnose a failure to step away from the narrow "campaigning mindset" (2021: 1), as the pandemic was regarded as irrelevant interlude. During his first press conference on the subject on 3 March, when he introduced a 'Coronavirus Action Plan', Prime Minister Johnson explicitly stated that drastic measures were not yet necessary, expressing confidence in the ability of the "fantastic NHS" (Johnson 2020a: 1) to manage the situation. He described the virus as "a mild disease from which [the majority of patients] will speedily and fully recover" (ibid.: 1). Consequently, no immediate countermeasures were recommended. At this stage, the virus appeared to be a problem requiring a response, but one that could be managed through established political routines and institutions, i.e. through politicisation.

By 16 March, however, the WHO had declared a pandemic and Johnson performed the first of numerous sudden U-turns during this crisis (cf. Holze 2023: 169ff.; Lilleker and Stoeckle 2021: 6). He presented the first public health guidelines advising infected individuals to minimise their movements, calling the situation "the worst public health crisis for a generation" (Johnson 2020c: 1). From this point on, he began his active securitization attempt by describing the virus and its potential consequences as a significant threat to the country. The issue had been moved from politicisation to securitization, with conventional political practices no longer being deemed adequate to address the problem (cf. Buzan et al. 1998: 29). Table 1 provides an overview of key events and significant policy changes in the UK during the period under examination or directly related to it.

Table 1: Overview of relevant dates and events in the development of the COVID-19 pandemic in the UK; data adapted from Aspinall (2021), Knock et al. (2021: 2) and Institute for Government (2022)

Date	Event or policy change
28 February	First infections within the UK
11 March	WHO declares pandemic
16 March	Movement restrictions announced
23 March	1st lockdown announced
26 March	Start of 1st lockdown
27 March	PM Johnson tests positive for the virus
5 April	PM Johnson admitted to hospital with COVID-19 infection
14 April	PM Johnson discharged from hospital
16 April	Introduction of the 'Five Tests' for lifting restrictions
19 April	Captain T. Moore raises money for NHS
22 May	Cummings scandal made public
23 June	Gradual relaxation of lockdown measures
29 June	Introduction of local lockdowns
14 August	Last nationwide lockdown restrictions lifted
14 September	Introduction of 'Rule of 6'
14 October	Introduction of tier system
31 October	2nd lockdown announced
5 November	Start 2nd lockdown
2 December	Lockdown restrictions lifted, tier system in place
8 December	First vaccinations against COVID-19 outside clinical trials in UK

This initial development reinforces the assertion that securitization is inherently a choice to address or ignore a particular issue made by the securitizing actor. Prime Minister Johnson's press conference of 16 March 2020 provides early evidence of this decision, in particular concerning the referent objects underlying his securitization of the COVID-19 pandemic. In his statement, Johnson remarks:

> "many more families are going to lose loved ones (...) this is now not just to attempt to contain the disease as far as possible, but to delay its spread and thereby minimise the suffering. If we delay the peak even by a few weeks, then our NHS will be in a stronger state (...), more beds are available and we'll have more time for medical research. We can also act to stretch the peak of the disease over a longer period so that our society is better able to cope."[1] (Johnson 2020c: 1)

He therefore proposes **two key referent objects**, namely the nation's health and the capacity of the NHS. Both fulfil the criteria for effective securitization outlined by Buzan et al. (cf. 1998: 31; see also section 2.2.3). The first – the rather abstract 'health' – refers to the medical status quo of the British nation, characterised by a population with a variety of individual health conditions yet devoid of any disease that poses a significant simultaneous threat to the majority. Naturally, their own health and survival, as well as that of family members and friends, are of paramount concern for each audience member. Thus, the prospect of widespread illness or death, particularly on a large scale, constitutes a distressing scenario for the public and satisfies the three requirements for a referent object.

Similarly, the second referent object – the National Health Service (NHS) – is widely regarded as a pillar of society and a source of national pride (cf. Burki 2018: 15f.). It has long been established as a respected and essential component of public well-being, a status reinforced during Johnson's Brexit campaign, where it was portrayed as a vital institution deserving of prioritised investment and protection. During this period, the NHS gained heightened symbolic importance, with its preservation and improved funding presented as a primary justification for leaving the European Union. The potential collapse of the NHS, which would render essential medical services unavailable, is universally recognised as catastrophic in the UK (cf. Campbell and Marsh 2020; Gregory and Campbell 2022; Roberts 2022). By presenting the COVID-19 pandemic

1 Austin (2023: 236) illustrates how this rhetoric was appropriated in a widely shared meme on Twitter (now X) in spring 2020. It references a line from the animated film Shrek, "Some of you may die, but that is a sacrifice I am willing to make", and employs it satirically to critique the underlying logic of Johnson's unempathetic discourse.

as an existential threat to these widely respected referent objects, Johnson successfully mobilised initial public support for extraordinary measures aimed at safeguarding them. This strategic alignment of valued referent objects with the urgency of the threat was instrumental in legitimising the securitization process.[2]

In turn, this prior collective consensus on the value of the NHS and public health facilitated Johnson's legitimacy as a **securitizing actor**. The person in this role must possess authority, credibility and the ability to speak on behalf of a broader collective, such as a nation, through an established position of power (cf. Buzan et al. 1998: 40f.). Johnson fulfils these criteria in his capacity as head of government, which grants him the institutional authority to define threats and propose exceptional measures. As an elected leader with a platform to address parliament and the public, he can present the pandemic as an impending existential crisis and propose extraordinary measures to protect vital referent objects, such as the NHS and national health. By leveraging his institutional legitimacy and alignment with shared societal values, Johnson is able to act as a persuasive advocate for securitization measures. While his speeches are typically directed at the general public to garner societal acceptance, the primary institutional mechanism for formalising securitization is parliamentary approval. This dual audience underscores the prime minister's role as both a representative of the collective and an authoritative voice.

For a successful securitization, the perceived **threat** must meet the criteria of being severe, dramatic in nature and capable of irreparably harming core societal principles or structures (cf. Buzan et al. 1998: 27). The issue must be

2 This initial support and trust in the government's approach proved to be short-lived. Boris Johnson sought to manage the crisis in a manner consistent with the persona he had cultivated over many years: that of an optimistic and strategically ambiguous, performative, anti-establishment "man of the people" characterised by populist affability (cf. Lilleker and Stoeckle 2021: 6; Paton 2022: 240). However, this communicative style was accompanied by a tendency to favour simple solutions despite the absence of sufficient knowledge to adequately address the crisis (cf. Spyridonidis et al. 2022: 684). As a result, the public grew increasingly critical of government's response, arguing that it was frequently unable "to understand scientific data, to postpone action for fear of overreaction, and to consistently underestimate the scale and pace of the challenge" (Horton 2023: 2277). Overall, Johnson's decisions were perceived as unclear, insufficiently grounded in scientific evidence, overly optimistic, and ultimately confusing to the public (cf. Spyridonidis et al. 2022: 688). Consequently, Johnson's approach was widely seen as contributing to an "egregiously poor outcome, the worst in Europe and one of the worst in the world" (Paton 2022: 238).

framed as an existential threat, asserting that a failure to address it would render all other concerns irrelevant as the survival of the audience itself would be at stake. In the case of the COVID-19 pandemic in Great Britain, the virus was initially securitized as an acute environmental threat, emphasising its sudden and catastrophic potential to overwhelm the NHS and endanger public health, both of which are critical pillars of British society. Over time, however, the discourse evolved from focusing on the immediate environmental crisis in a medical context to its broader socio-economic effects, such as the financial repercussions and public dissatisfaction with restrictive measures. This shift is indicative of a recurring pattern in securitization processes, where the urgency of acute environmental threats expands to encompass concerns in other sectors (cf. Buzan et al. 1998: 83). In securitizing COVID-19, Boris Johnson portrayed the virus as an existential threat with the potential to cause widespread illness and death, leading to the collapse of healthcare systems and, as a result, societal collapse. His securitizing move consistently conveys the urgent nature of the situation, arguing that without immediate and extraordinary measures, the NHS would be unable to maintain its functionality, resulting in irreparable harm to the nation.

The rhetorical structure of securitization, characterised by appeals to "urgency, survival and 'priority of action'" (Nyman 2012: 53), is therefore evident in Johnson's discourse surrounding the pandemic. However, these speech acts do not merely describe an existing security situation. Instead, they actively construct it themselves by successfully representing the virus as a massive security threat that requires immediate attention and action.

The **success** of a securitization attempt can only be evaluated retrospectively, based on whether the proposed extraordinary measures were implemented and broadly accepted. In the case of the UK's securitization of COVID-19, these criteria appear to have been met. The countermeasures introduced by Prime Minister Johnson, such as national lockdowns, were formally passed into law by the British Parliament and enforced as general behavioural guidelines. Despite multiple demonstrations, some comprising several thousand protesters (cf. Gayle 2020; Mercer 2020), and a minority of members of parliament – including opposition leader Keir Starmer – articulating concerns regarding specific measures (cf. Heffner 2020: 1), these expressions of dissent were limited and mostly directed at individual policies.

However, British **polls** conducted during the first year of the COVID-19 pandemic reveal a complex dynamic. After an initial "rally-round-the-flag effect" (Davies et al. 2021: 7), a relatively high proportion of the public expressed distrust of the government's ability to control the virus. The substantial, consistent support for the measures implemented by the government from April 2020 turned into distrust or neutrality for about 75% of Britons during the following months (cf. Davies et al. 2021: 6; Duffy 2020: 7). Nonetheless, throughout 2020, the overwhelming majority of the population attested to their adherence to all measures, including lockdowns and social distancing, either entirely or almost all the time (cf. Skinner and Garrett 2021: 1; Shepherd et al. 2023: 2). This widespread compliance suggests that the mobilisation of public and political support by Johnson's securitizing move was a success despite the poor performance with regard to public trust in the leadership. In presenting the pandemic as an existential threat requiring urgent and extraordinary action, the government succeeded despite the prevailing scepticism. It is important to note that the securitizing act was ongoing throughout the corpus period, with the primary focus shifting from convincing the public of the existential threat to emphasising the need for specific, timely interventions in response to the constantly evolving challenges, such as new virus variants or surges in infection rates.

This study primarily examines the illocutionary act. Consequently, the analysis focuses on the performative speech acts of the securitizing move itself. The empirical results over time, such as whether citizens supported the individual measures, are beyond the scope of this study.

5.2 Description of the corpus

The analysis encompasses the period between 3 March and 8 December 2020. These nine months represent the time between the first confirmed infections in the UK and the administration of the first vaccines against the virus in Great Britain. During this time, Prime Minister Boris Johnson delivered 46 speeches on the subject of the pandemic, which are documented in this corpus. The majority of these statements pertain to the ongoing crisis in England, as the other three constituent parts of the United Kingdom – Scotland, Wales and Northern Ireland – are led by First Ministers, who are responsible for making their own decisions in matters of health.

Overall, the dataset comprises:

- 36 statements made at press conferences,
- four statements delivered in the House of Commons,

- two articles in newspapers, i.e. the *Mail on Sunday* (7 May 2020) and the *Belfast Telegraph* (13 August 2020),
- one transcribed video message,
- one Economy Speech (30 June 2020) as delivered in Dudley,
- one speech at the Global Vaccine Summit, and
- one speech to the United Nations General Assembly.

The initial statement was issued on 3 March 2020, while the final statement included in this analysis is the address delivered on 2 December 2020, as no other recorded statements were documented until the administration of the first vaccines against SARS-CoV-2 six days later. Figure 1 shows the number of press statements per month in the *JPanC20*.

Figure 1: Number of monthly press statements by Prime Minister Boris Johnson in the JPanC20; the December figure is not comparable to the other months in absolute terms as the dataset only includes two days for this month

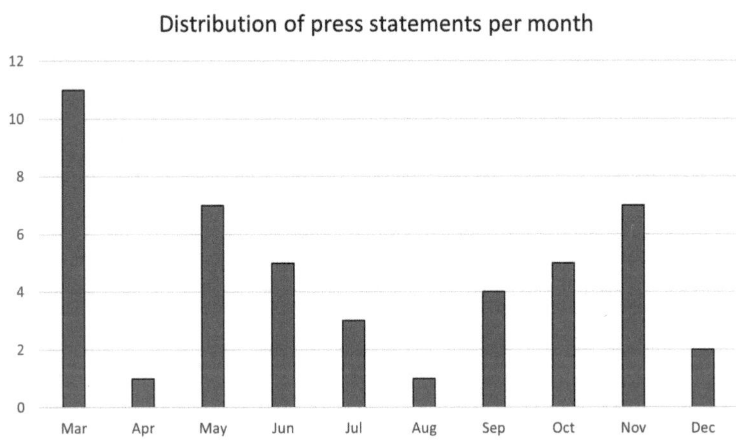

All publications are in the form that is displayed on the official government website for press statements, www.gov.uk/search/news-and-communication s (cf. Government of the United Kingdom 2024), with no alterations to punctuation or other typographical conventions. Press releases containing paraphrased or partial quotations of Johnson's words have been excluded, as have joint statements with other actors, such as the President of the European Commission (cf. Johnson and von der Leyen 2020). Similarly, press statements or interviews by other government officials, such as the Chancellor of the Duchy of Lancaster or the Foreign Secretary, have not been included in this corpus as they do not necessarily reflect the prime minister's narrative of threat.

5.3 Corpus Analysis

The resulting *JPanC20* consists of 56,349 tokens, i.e. the absolute number of words in the dataset, and 4,632 types, i.e. the number of different words in the dataset, which results in a **type-token-ratio** (TTR)[3] of 8.2%. This value is rather low, which points to a lower lexical diversity in the dataset and a relatively high frequency of repetitions and formulaic speech (cf. Cheng 2012: 63). As the prime minister is talking about one single topic – the pandemic and its ramifications in the form of developments, measures and consequences – this first part is not surprising. The second element, the formulaic speech, is explained to some extent by the inherent structure of press conferences and statements in the House of Commons, with repetitive greetings and particular modes of addressing the audience, as well as being due to the content of the press statements. Following a distinctive structure may provide the audience with a sense of familiarity, thereby instilling a reassuring feeling of control. Furthermore, considering that the prime minister's task is to announce measures such as lockdown restrictions or different tiers, it is very probable that he would engage in formulaic utterances, often using the same phrases and words.

5.3.1 Word frequencies

The content of the dataset can be characterised in more detail by looking at the word frequencies. This section of the analysis was conducted with the program *AntConc*.

3 The Type-Token-Ratio is defined as the quotient of the number of types divided by the number of tokens. This measurement is expressed as a value between 0 and 1, in this case: $\frac{4633}{56349} = 0.082 = 8.2\%$. A higher percentage signifies a higher linguistic diversity within the corpus as it offers a relatively high number of different types (cf. Depala 2023: 1; Cheng 2012: 63).

The prevalence of articles, conjunctions and prepositions characteristic of the English language is reflected in this list, given that 'the' with 3,078 occurrences, 'and' with 2,332 and 'to' with 2,168 are the three most frequent words. In this initial stage of the analysis, function words are excluded through the creation of a **stop list**, a collection of high-frequency words that provide minimal information as they are not directly related to the content dimension of the corpus. Such lists are often utilised to enable a focused examination of the primary topics and qualitative findings (cf. Hvitfeldt and Silge 2022: 37f.). They typically comprise frequent function words inherent to the English language, including definite and indefinite articles, prepositions, conjunctions, determiners, qualifiers and question words (cf. Wynne 2008: 729; Doyle 2023: 1). At this stage of the analysis, the three most frequent words in the corpus, 'the', 'and' and 'to', do not provide useful information that contributes to an understanding of the corpus or aids in answering the research questions. Instead, they act as an impediment when analysing the data with automated software like *AntConc*, particularly when attempting to identify patterns, because of their ubiquity. For this reason, a stop list excludes these words from the 100 most frequent words, thus allowing a focus on the more semantically substantial elements of the text and, in turn, enhancing the precision and efficacy of the analytical process. In contrast to the conventional approach to stop lists (cf. Burns 2018: 4), this analysis incorporates pronouns as well as auxiliary and modal verbs, which may prove useful in gaining deeper insight into the *JPanC20*. The stop list is shown in figure A1 in the appendix[4]. The adjusted list of the remaining 57 most frequent words in the 100 most frequent words in the *JPanC20* is depicted in table 2 below.

4 All figures titled A(*number*) are found in the appendix.

Table 2: Adapted list of the 100 most frequent words in the JPanC20; stop list applied; sorted by absolute frequency

Rank	Word	Frequ. (abs.)	Rank	Word	Frequ. (abs.)	Rank	Word	Frequ. (abs.)
4	we	1559	44	nhs	160	71	testing	103
10	will	685	46	been	151	72	down	99
11	i	661	50	country	148	73	take	98
15	is	649	52	work	136	74	coron-avirus	97
16	are	597	53	must	134	75	lives	97
20	have	567	54	want	134	76	should	97
22	our	499	55	covid	130	77	home	94
24	it	442	56	measures	125	79	no	92
25	be	429	60	us	124	80	together	92
26	you	346	61	uk	123	81	other	91
30	people	320	62	your	122	82	every	90
32	can	314	63	time	118	83	going	89
33	virus	231	64	local	117	84	today	88
34	more	202	65	know	114	85	t	87
35	has	194	66	new	112	86	disease	85
36	s	190	67	would	112	89	tests	83
38	their	185	68	need	108	90	am	82
40	they	180	69	get	105	92	govern-ment	80
42	do	167	70	way	104	93	next	80

A total of 20 **verbs** are included in this list. It produces the following 13 verbs when lemmatised: be, have, can, do, work, must, want, know, need, get, take, should, go. The two most frequent verbs, 'be' and 'have', are essential for forming various tenses in English, given their function both as auxiliary verbs and lexical verbs stating or describing something or expressing possession. Thus, they typically occur in very high ranks. They might also already allude to a high frequency of assertives in the dataset that state new developments, explain something or give information. Similarly, the modal verbs 'can', 'must' and 'should' are used to express modality, including possibilities, necessities or obligations. Their high frequency in combination with semi-modals like 'want' and 'need' suggests that the corpus comprises a significant number of expressions of ability, necessity, duty or desire. This finding initially gives the impression that the dataset may contain a considerable number of directives. However, a closer look at 'must', a verb highly probable for this category and ranked 53rd on the frequency list, shows that this first interpretation is incorrect. The most frequent collocate on the left side of the modal verb, which occurs 134 times in the corpus, is the pronoun 'we', with over 85 cases. The combination 'we+must' is therefore a typical example within this dataset. In some instances, it functions as a commissive speech act directed towards the government (cf. Johnson 2020n: 1), whereas in other cases, it represents a reference to the nation. This use is often found in assertives, e.g. in the following explanation: "we must make sure that any measures we take do not force the reproduction rate of the disease (…) back up over one, so that we have the kind of exponential growth we were facing a few weeks ago" (Johnson 2020t: 2). Although the differentiation is sometimes subtle and challenging, this use of the modal verb rather points to a greater presence of commissive and assertive speech acts instead of directives. Moreover, there are only 43 instances of commands utilising 'you+must' or 'you+need to', rendering this speech act directed at the public a moderately relevant, yet not overwhelmingly significant occurrence.[5] Instead, Johnson's collaborative approach is emphasised once again by his focus on messages containing the pronoun in the first person plural. However, the frequent discussion of possible action, recommendations and a certain position of authority may already be inferred from this list.

---

5 In contrast, the commissive 'I+must' occurs 21 times, approximately one third of which is an emphasis ('I+must+stress/emphasise'). Contextualised, these functions act as reassuring or warning speech acts. Nine instances are cautionary utterances ('I+must+be clear/level with you' (7) and 'I+must+say/be frank' (2)), three were identified as directive speech acts ('I+must+ask the public' (2) and 'I+must+ give an instruction'). The last two occurrences, both declarative utterances, present Johnson as forced by circumstances: "I must do what is necessary" (Johnson 2020ac: 2) with regard to the second lockdown, and "I must now proceed with moving Greater Manchester (…) to the Very High alert level" (Johnson 2020ai: 2). None of these commit Johnson personally to do anything, unlike the personalised directive 'you+must'. 'I+need to' is not found in the corpus.

By contrast, the verbs 'work', 'know', 'get', 'take' and 'go' are basic high-frequency verbs in English that are used to describe common actions or mental states. Their mid-range position in the list implies that the corpus comprises everyday actions or states of being. It can be concluded that the aforementioned terms may be indicative of the texts' focus on general activities, personal needs and common experiences.

The second most frequent word is the verb 'will', which illustrates the speaker's emphasis on the future, including inevitable or planned actions. Similarly, the bigram 'we+will' is the second most frequent, predominantly paired with 'continue to' (17 instances), 'be able to' (16) and 'get through' (10). The additional appearance of 'going' at rank 83 on this frequency list, functioning as the first component of 'going+to', reinforces this idea. This node co-occurs mostly with 'do it' and 'beat it' in postposition, which imply a notion of achieving results and overcoming obstacles. When considered together, they suggest that the expression of planned action or anticipated developments occupies a significant position within the corpus.

The **pronouns** 'we', 'I', 'our' and 'you' are among the ten most frequent words and suggest the existence of an audience or group to which the speaker belongs. It can be observed that 'we' and 'our' are used with greater frequency than 'I' and 'my'. Indeed, the latter is only encountered 33 times across the entire dataset and, as a result, does not appear in table 2. This finding leads to the conclusion that the focus seems to be on the community rather than on the speaker or the individual. While the most common trigram, 'I want to', may initially appear to indicate a typical self-centred expression of desire on the part of the speaker, a more detailed examination of its object suggests otherwise. The most common 4-gram with the pronoun in the first person singular is 'I want to+thank', found 27 times, which supports the idea that the author is more focused on acknowledging the contributions of others than on expressing personal desires. These utterances mostly address the nation, e.g.: "I want to thank you[,] the people of this country" (Johnson 2020g: 1). This result also reflects the significance of the speech act 'thank' for the prime minister's communication.

However, once again, it is not evident which entity is being referenced by the plural pronouns, as 'we' could signify either the British citizens or the government. Consequently, a more detailed examination of each subsequent verb is necessary, which will be incorporated into the subsequent analysis of speech acts. Moreover, a detailed examination of the most prevalent trigrams with this pronoun reveals a dual temporal focus within the dataset. With 26 instances each, the trigrams 'we+are now' and 'we+will be' display Johnson's concern with the status quo and his efforts to direct the course of future events. Similarly, despite its apparent directness, the pronoun 'you' can be interpreted as addressing multiple audiences, among them members of parliament, all citizens, the press or more specific groups, such as Mancunians (cf. Johnson 2020r: 2).

A notable **cluster** in this frequency list are terms pertaining to the **medical crisis**, including 'virus', 'nhs', 'covid', 'measures', 'testing', 'coronavirus', 'lives', 'disease' and 'tests'. They revolve around the ongoing public health crisis related to the SARS-CoV-2 pandemic, as demonstrated by 'virus', 'covid', 'coronavirus' and 'disease'. The term 'nhs' establishes a distinct UK-centric perspective, with a likely emphasis on the role of the healthcare infrastructure in pandemic management. An emphasis on mitigating and preventive measures might be inferred from the nodes 'measures' and 'testing', whereas 'lives' and 'disease' appear to be associated with the human toll of the pandemic. In combination with 'uk', 'government' and 'home', this cluster indicates a corpus pertaining to official pronouncements by a British government official.

Similarly, an additional cluster appears to establish a particularly **patriotic tone** within the list of the most frequently occurring words. Expressions such as 'we', 'our', 'people', 'country', 'uk', 'home', 'together', and to a lesser extent also 'lives', 'every' and 'government', evoke a frame of unity and nation. These terms convey a sense of inclusivity, community and shared identity, frequently expressing sentiments of solidarity, patriotism and national pride. The use of terms such as 'lives', 'every' and 'government' strengthens this tone by indicating that the discussion is focused on serious matters that impact the entire nation or population. This approach has probably been designed to unite the nation by emphasising shared values and collective goals, thus fostering a sense of group cohesion, possibly to encourage unity in the face of challenges and legitimise decisions made by the leaders.

5.3.2 Keywords

An examination of keywords can assist in determining whether these words are naturally common in an English corpus. Table 3 provides an overview of the 20 most characteristic **keywords** in comparison to the reference corpus, the *BE06* (cf. Baker 2009). The list is organised in descending order of keyness, as measured in Log-Likelihood.

Table 3: List of the 20 most characteristic keywords in the JPanC20 in comparison to the BE06; sorted by keyness (Log-Likelihood); frequencies given in absolute numbers

Rank	Word	Frequ. (JPanC20)	Frequ. (BE06)	Key-ness	Rank	Word	Frequ. (JPanC20)	Frequ. (BE06)	Key-ness
1	we	1559	3406	3384	11	vaccine	64	3	351
2	virus	231	20	1220	12	restric-tions	77	23	347
3	will	685	2160	1124	13	Lock-down	65	6	341
4	our	499	1358	921	14	are	597	4491	319
5	covid	130	0	764	15	have	567	4176	316
6	nhs	160	93	617	16	and	2332	28069	312
7	coron-avirus	97	0	570	17	now	279	1321	303
8	people	320	1340	399	18	country	148	354	299
9	mea-sures	125	131	394	19	speaker	68	23	299
10	testing	103	79	364	20	tests	83	70	284

Four groups of keywords can be identified. The first comprises three **names for SARS-CoV-19**: virus, covid and coronavirus. Two of these are absent from the *BE06*, as the name of the virus had not been established prior to the first infections with this particular pathogen in 2019. The third node, 'virus', appears over 100 times more in the target corpus, with 321 absolute instances compared to only 20 in the *BE06*. This imbalance results in a normalised frequency[6] of 4,099 in the corpus of press statements by Boris Johnson as compared to 19 in the *BE06* corpus, which equates to a frequency approximately 205 times greater. This finding identifies the topic as one of considerable significance, which seems an accurate reflection of the subject matter of the press statements under discussion.

The next keyword group is closely linked to the first. Extending the above focus on names for the virus, it contains words associated with **pandemic-contextual terms**. This cluster consists of the following six terms: measures,

6 Per 1,000,000 words

testing, vaccine, restrictions, lockdown and tests. Without naming it explicitly, they reference the virus via contextual clues as they are all closely related to the political management of the health crisis. This is evidenced by their significant overrepresentation in comparison to the *BE06*. Although not uncommon in pre-pandemic discourse, their likelihood numbers range from 394 to 284, suggesting a significantly more prominent position in the target corpus compared to the *BE06*. Several of these terms for a medical crisis are therefore uncommon in everyday British English and considerably more prevalent within the special corpus. Whereas the absolute number of 'measures' is in a similar range in both corpora, the expressions 'vaccines', 'restrictions' and 'lockdown' occur 50 to 60 times more frequently than in the entire *BE06*. This statistically significant difference leads to normalised frequencies of 1,135 per 1,000,000 tokens in comparison to five for 'vaccine*', as well as 1,366 as opposed to 23 for 'restrictions', and 1,153 as compared to six for 'lockdown'. The normalised frequency for the node 'measures', although comparable in total numbers, multiplies by the factor 17, with 130 in the *BE06* and 2,218 in the *JPanC20*. The considerable relevance of these keywords for the analysis corpus is therefore evident, pointing to measures that counter the crisis.

The third cluster of keywords consists of the pronouns 'we' and 'our', in addition to the nouns 'people' and 'country', and the verbs 'are' and 'have'. They are unified by a common understanding of **community** and a shared set of values. The pronoun 'we', ranked first on the keyness table in table 3, highlights its significantly higher relevance in the corpus under examination. Its normalised frequency is 27,667, which amounts to about eight times that of the *BE06* (3,380). The possessive 'our' sees an increase by a factor of 6.5 from 1,348 in the corpus of British English to 8,855 in the *JPanC20*. The distinctiveness of these two pronouns may be attributed to a communicative style that aims to foster an inclusive and collective identity by addressing a group to which the speaker himself belongs. The use of the nouns 'people' and 'country', with their respective keyness rates of 399 and 299, highlights this communal aspect. The former has a normalised frequency of 5,679 times per 1,000,000 tokens in the *JPanC20*, which is over four times the normalised occurrence in the BE06 (1,330). The contrast is even starker with 'country', which shows a normalised frequency approximately 7.5 times greater in the *JPanC20* with 2,626, as compared to 351 in the *BE06*. Additionally, the verbs 'are' and 'have', ranked here in positions 14 and 15, exhibit a smaller but still significant gap in value, with a normalised presence multiplied by 2.3 and 2.4 respectively in favour of the corpus under examination. This third cluster of keywords centring around community and shared values illustrates Johnson's evident emphasis on these elements by situating the discourse within a national context, thereby underscoring the intention to unite the community under a shared banner of citizenship or nationality.

The final group of keywords is not closely related in terms of content but rather serves to **situate an utterance in its context**. It consists of three expressions: 'nhs', 'speaker' and 'now'. The first of them, the abbreviation 'nhs' for National Health Service, is a uniquely British term. Its position in table 3 demonstrates its importance for the government during the crisis. Despite the fact that it appears 92 times per 1,000,000 words in the *BE06*, which already signals a smaller but evident relevance for the culture behind this English variety, its normalised frequency of 2,839 for the target corpus demonstrates its status as one of the key priorities and cornerstones of the government's strategy in the context of the crisis.

The word 'speaker', usually in the combination 'Mr+Speaker' (62 hits), alludes to the nature of some of the press statements, as they are transcripts of speeches given in the House of Commons. There, it is common to address the speaker in this way several times per contribution. This keyword therefore situates the corpus in a parliamentary context, highlighting Johnson's position within the government, which is demonstrated by a normalised frequency of 1207, as compared to 23 in the *BE06*. This results in a keyness rate of 299, illustrating that while it is slightly less significant comparatively, it remains highly relevant for the *JPanC20*.

Lastly, the use of 'now', with a likelihood of 303, underscores the irrefutable connection between the utterances and a specific period. Johnson frequently employs this deictic expression to report on the present circumstances and ongoing actions, thereby emphasising the preliminary figures and the respective provisional assessment. It occurs 279 times in the *JPanC20*, compared to 1,321 occurrences in the *BE06*, which translates into a position as the 17th most characteristic keyword in table 3. Its high placement serves to illustrate the cautious manner in which Johnson announces interim measures and temporary plans, which are contingent upon the further development of the crisis. Its high frequency can also be explained by its potential to appear in all five speech act categories.

The **results** of the corpus analysis indicate that the most prevalent words and expressions in the corpus place a strong emphasis on the concepts of community and national unity. These linguistic patterns suggest that the communication strategy is designed to emotionally engage the public and emphasise collective responsibility in order to motivate cooperative behaviour. In order to gain a deeper understanding of Johnson's strategy in securitizing the pandemic, it is necessary to examine the underlying speech acts in closer detail as it is not merely the content of his statements but also their stylistic nuances that shape the actions he realises through language. The following analysis will therefore focus on the illocutionary acts employed during the crisis communication.

5.4 Speech Act Analysis

Figure 2: Speech act category percentages within the JPanC20

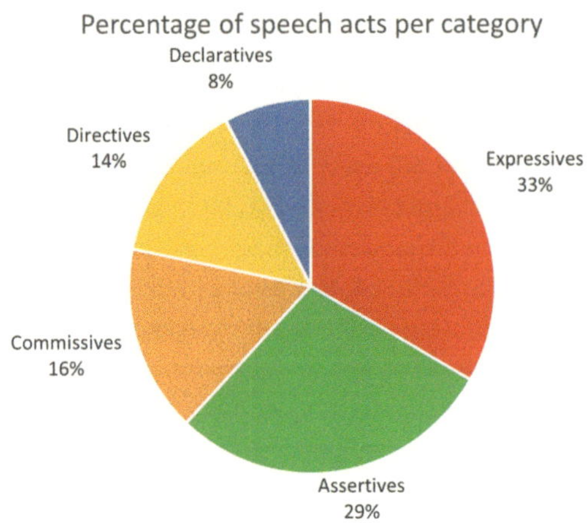

Altogether, 1,271 individual speech acts were coded. This results in a speech act distribution in which expressives represent the largest category at 33%. The next most frequent category is assertive speech acts with 29%, whereas commissives and directives account for 16% and 14% of the corpus respectively, as shown in figure 2. The category of declarative utterances represents only 8% of the total dataset, making it the smallest category. Johnson therefore tends to place a particular emphasis on the first category, which illustrate "an emotive connection between the addresser and the addressee or the addresser and the described situation" (Marsen and Ali-Chand 2022: 8). Figure 2 shows the distribution of speech act categories in this dataset.

These categories are then further subdivided into subcategories.

Searle's five categories (assertives, expressives, commissives, directives and declaratives) are further subdivided into subcategories, which in turn contain individual speech acts, which are made up by the single utterances. Table A1 in the appendix visualises this differentiation. Marsen and Ali-Chand's initial classification of subcategories (cf. 2022: 8) has been adapted to the characteristics of the *JPanC20* and modified inductively. In particular, they proposed the two expressive subcategories of sympathy and gratitude, which were subsequently inductively supplemented by ten additional subcategories. In regard to assertive speech acts, the concept of the subcategory 'describe' was derived from the aforementioned article and subsequently divided into three constituent elements, which were then complemented by four additional subcategories. The commissive subcategories 'threaten', 'warn' and 'promise action' have been created in a refined adaptation of those proposed by Marsen and Ali-Chand (2022). While the first two correspond to the respective speech act, the latter is now separated into six individual speech acts due to the characteristic features of this corpus. Moreover, the directive subcategories 'command' and 'request' have both been further subdivided in this work, and two additional subcategories, 'motivate' and 'advise the public', have been introduced. Lastly, only one type of declarative was described in the 2022 article. This has been differentiated into three subcategories for the purpose of this research.

5.4.1 Expressive speech acts

A total of 424 occurrences of expressives have been identified. On average, they encompass 220 characters including spaces. The smallest expressive is "So thank you" (Johnson 2020a6: 3) with only 13 characters, the shortest individual speech act in the entire dataset, whereas the largest expressive contains 1,468 characters (cf. figure A4 and A5).

Expressive speech acts have been divided into 12 subcategories, predominantly called after the emotion they convey. Expressing 'gratitude', 'sympathy', 'pride' and 'anger' are further subdivided into several different speech acts, whereas 'confidence', 'caution', 'hope', 'relief', 'grief', 'impatience', 'hedging/deflecting' and 'personal experience' each stand for an individual speech act with the same name. Of all expressive speech acts, 97% were found to express feelings. The three largest single emotions are gratitude with 31% or 131 instances, sympathy/understanding with 20% or 87 instances, and pride with 64 instances, which amounts to 15%. All other feelings occur less than 50 times.

In addition to the subcategories denoting feelings, two minor subcategories have been identified within the dataset. The first of them is 'hedging/deflecting'. It refers to ten instances of Boris Johnson evading a direct response regarding specific figures or dates or, alternatively, emphasising that the information he has just presented is subject to change depending on the evolving circumstances. It has been included in this category because these statements are connected to a feeling of uncertainty or indecisiveness. As he avoids stating facts, these utterances cannot be classified as assertives. Similarly, his refusal to commit to specific actions precludes the possibility of classifying them as commissive speech acts.

The second of these subcategories, 'personal experience', occurs four times. In these instances, the prime minister discusses his personal experience as a patient diagnosed with the virus, offering his impressions and feelings. Consequently, these emotional expressions have been classified as instances of expressive speech acts.

Figure 3: Subcategory percentages within the category 'Expressives' in the JPanC20[7]

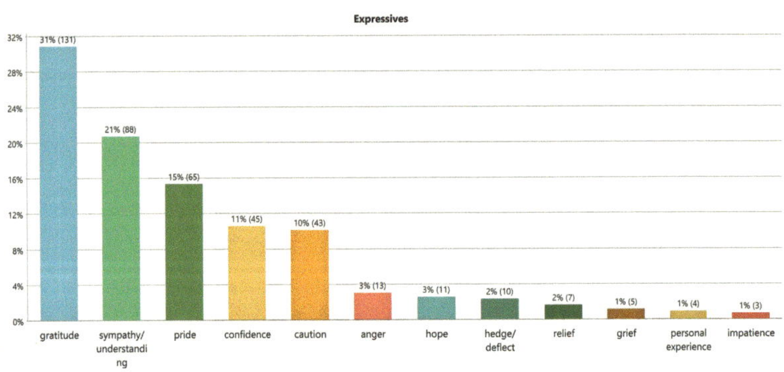

7 All diagrams showing speech act percentages in chapter 6 were made by the author with tools from the software MAXQDA, Version 2024.4.1 (cf. Verbi 2024).

Figure 3 gives an overview of the distribution of speech acts in the category 'Expressives'.[8]

5.4.1.1 Gratitude

The most frequently occurring subcategory in the category of expressive speech acts is that of showing gratitude, with 131 instances. Its frequency makes it one of the key features of Boris Johnson's communication strategy. It consists of the two elements 'acknowledging others' and 'thanking'. The exact distribution of speech acts in the subcategory 'gratitude' is shown in figure 4.

Figure 4: Speech act distribution within the subcategory 'gratitude' in the JPanC20

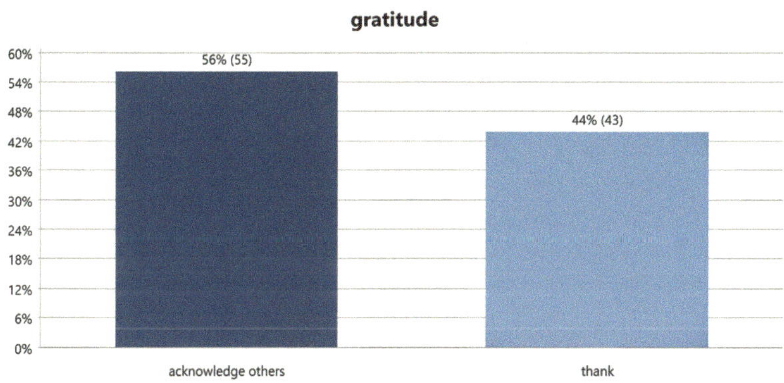

Utterances **acknowledging others** were identified on 88 occasions. This speech act differs from thanking in that it highlights the individual's considerable efforts or the outcome of these, implying, although not explicitly stating, an underlying expression of gratitude or respect. In particular, Johnson acknowledges several senior doctors or scientists as advisers in 32 cases, including Sir Patrick Vallance, Chief Scientific Adviser, and Sir Christopher Whitty, Chief Medical Officer. The second group of addressees are other politicians, such as then-chancellor Rishi Sunak, Baroness Harding, who acted as

8 Expressive speech acts are predominantly designated according to the following structure: "express *emotion*". For the sake of brevity, they are only labelled with the respective emotion in the diagrams, with the prior "express" omitted.

head of the *Test and Trace* programme[9], and local leaders in hotspot areas (23 hits), with whom he coordinated emergency measures. NHS care workers, police, security guards and teachers are acknowledged four times, as are ordinary citizens, for their patience and compliance with the restrictions. He applauds the nation's teachers on three occasions, while other workers, such as employees in the food industry, transport workers, doctors, refuse collectors, cleaners, civil and public servants, engineers or postal workers, are mentioned only once or twice. Similarly, the efforts of the four British nations as well as the dedication of British companies are highlighted three times, in both cases emphasising their efficacy in the face of challenging circumstances. In autumn – towards the end of the dataset – the military and the Vaccines Task Force are mentioned four times. During this period, the implementation of an immunisation programme was imminent, with vaccine administration to be conducted by the armed forces. Their acknowledgement reflects the government's new priorities at that time.

Besides scientists or doctors and fellow politicians, Johnson is therefore mentioning different groups from the British public and recognising their contributions to the collective effort. His main focus seems to be on acknowledging the scientific advisers and politicians with whom he is working closely to draft response measures to current developments. The slightly higher number of medical personnel and scientists named (32 cases) indicates that the situation is being treated as a medical emergency. This figure increases by a factor of 7.75 when shifting the focus to his personal advisers, who are mentioned in almost every press statement in the examined period. This may be attributed to the fact that some of them frequently share the stage with the prime minister, which presents him with the opportunity to express his appreciation of them as a polite gesture. However, this figure can also be attributed to their direct influence on pivotal decisions and strategies during this period of crisis. Johnson

9 Advertised in May by the prime minister as "world-beating" (Johnson 2020m: 3), the Test and Trace programme soon proved to be overwhelmed during the summer months. Nevertheless, Johnson insisted that it was fully functional until November (cf. Reuters 2020: 1).This blunder was "assessed as a £37 billion failure" (Paton 2021: 1979, see also Holze 2023: 171f.). Paton (2022) also sarcastically remarked on the lack of consequences given the high number of cases traced: It "seemed odd that there were too many cases to allow community testing to be possible, yet also too few to justify lockdown" (Paton 2022: 239). Ultimately, he described the programme as being more like "Alice in Wonderland than 'world beating'" (ibid.: 1976).

appears to regard their expertise as a crucial element in the effective management of the situation and the overarching objective of ensuring the well-being of the nation.

Other professions seem to be credited in a rather enumerative manner, as they appear in lists of acknowledgements without a detailed description of their contribution or its effects, e.g. in Johnson's article in the *Mail on Sunday* (cf. Johnson 2020p). Teachers, however, are typically mentioned separately and with an additional comment on their effort, rather than being included in longer lists. This may be due to the government's explicit objective of keeping schools open. One example is the following statement from 24 May: "this [new measure of opening schools] comes after a constructive period of consultation with schools, teachers and unions" (Johnson 2020q: 2). The police are not included in the lists either. Instead, they are referenced separately in the context of restrictions that must be enforced. Overall, the prime minister acknowledges a large number of groups and individuals as important in times of crisis, which suggests an inclusive approach. He not only focuses on emergency responders but also on people whose daily contributions are crucial to mitigating the broader social and economic impact of the crisis. This demonstrates an understanding that effective crisis management and, ultimately, recovery from this crisis necessitates coordination across numerous sectors and the dedication of a vast number of individuals. For the audience, this gesture of recognition and appreciation fosters a sense of unity and shared endeavour, which might help to maintain their motivation and resilience.

One third of speech acts in the subcategory 'gratitude' are instances in which Johnson explicitly **thanks** others. The primary addressee of this is the British public, whom he mentions on 20 occasions. He mainly commends citizens for their everyday sacrifices and efforts, which are deemed essential to minimise the virus reproduction numbers. For this speech act, he employs statements such as "I want to thank you[,] the people of this country[,] for the sheer grit and guts you have shown and are continuing to show" (Johnson 2020l: 1), or "we are passing through the peak (...) thanks to your forbearance, your good sense[,] your altruism[,] your spirit of community[,] thanks to our collective national resolve" (ibid.). His choice of words shows a profound appreciation that situates individual actions within the broader context of a heroic narrative of progress, to which everybody contributes. He addresses them directly with the second-person plural pronoun and in this example specifies, "you[,] the people of this country", thereby making the statement and the expression of gratitude more personal and immediate. This approach not only acknowledges the contributions of individuals in the community, as indicated by the elements "your forbearance[,] your good sense[,] your altruism", but also highlights their efforts, conveying a sense of collective pride and purpose with the subsequent elements "your spirit of community" and "our collective national resolve". In the last part, Johnson incorporates himself into the addressed group, thus shifting from the pure act of thanking the nation for their contributions to the connected act of praising the audience and himself. By employing the pronoun in the first person plural, he draws attention not only to the determination and resilience of the public but also to his own efforts and those of his administration, thereby suggesting that these qualities were instrumental in reaching this point. His choice of words suggests a heroic frame that places individual activities into the wider context of a battle narrative, resembling the rhetoric of a wartime speech (cf. Rawlinson 2020: 1; see also Musolff 2022). This contextualisation of individual actions serves to enhance public morale and emphasises the crucial role of individual and collective actions in crisis management. Furthermore, it also illustrates the prime minister's strategy of using gratitude to foster a sense of unity and shared purpose among the British people.

Besides these expressions of gratitude not linked to specific events, there are also instances of issuing a 'thank you' for particular occasions, for example the British Mother's Day on 22 March 2020. By listing specific actions such as calling, Facetiming or Skyping one's mother, the prime minister expresses his gratitude that people chose these individual actions to replace the traditional visit on this day, which was prohibited by lockdown regulations. He added his understanding of the challenges and emotions posed by the restrictions on a day of celebration, stressing the fact that collective action has the potential to amplify the effect of the restrictive measures (cf. Johnson 2020h: 1). He thus situates the actions of each citizen within a narrative of collaboration, for which he expresses his gratitude. By acknowledging the emotional difficulty of the demanded behaviour and explicitly thanking them for it, Johnson's words may serve as intrinsic motivation for citizens to persevere in their efforts and continue to minimise social contact.

The *JPanC20* contains seven instances of thanking teachers and head teachers. This sentiment is observed consistently throughout the entire period of the dataset, providing insight into one of the government's primary objectives during the pandemic: maintaining the operational status of educational institutions. This is almost equalled by the number of thanks addressed to NHS staff, including doctors, who are not referenced separately. There are five expressions of gratitude for their invaluable work, which are solidified by the six grateful mentions of medical volunteers, including the citizens of Liverpool. These individuals demonstrated their commitment by participating in vaccine trials or returning to active duty after retirement to support their fellow healthcare professionals in hospitals. Johnson repeatedly refers to the National Health Service (NHS) as an indispensable component of British national identity. Especially during and after his own infection with the virus in March and April 2020, he highlights the "amazing NHS staff" (Johnson 2020k: 1) and thanks them explicitly for their work.[10] Moreover, he identifies it as an imperative priority for the government to navigate with caution in order to avoid overwhelming the healthcare system (cf. Johnson 2020v: 1). By explicitly acknowledging the contributions of medical professionals, including doctors, nurses and hospital staff, he underscores their vital role in addressing the medical emergency. Simultaneously, the prime minister mentions the sacrifices and working conditions of the volunteers, emphasising their need for assistance from the wider community, which can contribute by maintaining social distance. Expressing gratitude to the NHS volunteers is primarily used to commend their altruism and "stepping up" (Johnson 2020l: 1) in a time of crisis. It is frequently accompanied by a success statement, such as the low infection rates or the promising progress in vaccine development, in a demonstration that their efforts and hard work are worthwhile.

Similar to the NHS volunteers, essential workers in areas like food production or public transportation are addressed four times. Due to the format of press statements, Johnson also thanks the audience four times, which always occurs at the beginning or end of the speech. His expressions of gratitude to others play a relatively minor role, with one or two mentions over the course of the ten months in the evaluation period. They encompass other members of government (two), the military (two), leading national scientists who were thanked after giving input at the press conferences (two), business owners and local politicians, as well as Bill and Melinda Gates for their contributions to global vaccine research, which took place in the context of a *Global Vaccine Summit* in June 2020. Some of these recipients of gratitude have already been refer-

10 Another expression of gratitude for the contribution of NHS workers was the weekly 'Clap for Our Carers' initiative (cf. Addley 2020), a social movement that saw Britons expressing their appreciation for essential workers, particularly those in the NHS, through clapping at their doorsteps from March until May 2020. Johnson references these events in the dataset (cf. Johnson 2020k: 1).

enced in the first element of this subcategory, 'acknowledging others'. In contrast to this earlier mention, the instances in this second segment of the subcategory provide a summary of occasions where they are not only acknowledged but also explicitly thanked for their contributions.

Overall, the high number of expressions of gratitude and acknowledgement fosters a sense of unity and solidarity by helping to bring society together through a common goal in times of difficulty. The importance of collaboration is highlighted, which facilitates greater inter-sectoral cooperation and mutual support. Expressing gratitude can have the effect of enhancing the morale of the general public, particularly of those mentioned, motivating them to continue their efforts since these are perceived as being impactful and valued by the government and community. The frequent mention of thanking citizens, rather than specific professions or smaller groups of people, demonstrates the government's belief that the situation requires the efforts of the whole country and can only be resolved through joint efforts.

5.4.1.2 Sympathy/understanding

Within the category 'expressives', speech acts showing **understanding or sympathy** account for 20% or 87 instances. They constitute the second subcategory, which is further divided into the four elements 'show understanding', 'sympathise', 'express regret' and 'apologise'. Figure 5 illustrates the distribution of speech acts in this subcategory.

Figure 5: Speech act distribution within the subcategory 'sympathy/understanding' in the JPanC20

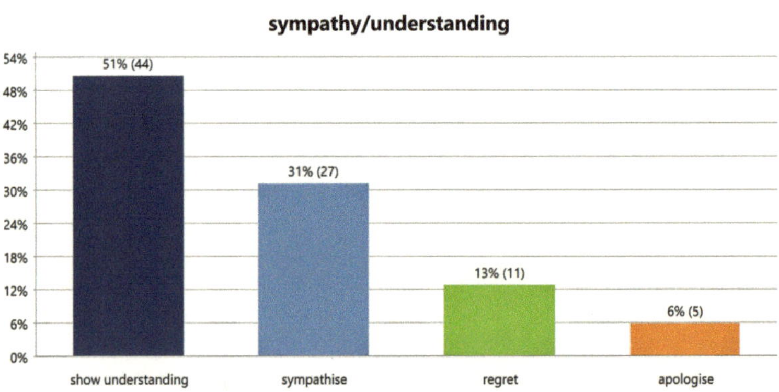

In 44 instances, Boris Johnson demonstrates an **understanding** of citizens' sentiments, predominantly regarding the challenges they are facing in adapting to new restrictions (cf. Johnson 2020ac: 1), their frustration with these measures (cf. Johnson 2020s: 2) and regarding their concerns about potential personal consequences (cf. Johnson 2020i: 2). He frequently offers compassionate comments validating feelings of frustration or being overwhelmed, such as "I know it is tough" (Johnson 2020l: 3) and demonstrates his profound understanding of the difficult situation that citizens find themselves in by providing extensive illustrations. One particular example is his statement from 27 April:

> "I know how hard and how stressful it has been to give up even temporarily,[] those ancient and basic freedoms[,] not seeing friends[,] not seeing loved ones[,] working from home[,] managing the kids[,] worrying about your job and your firm[,] so let me say directly also to British business[,] to the shopkeepers[,] to the entrepreneurs[,] to the hospitality sector[,] to everyone on whom our economy depends[,] I understand your impatience[.]"[11] (Johnson 2020l: 2)

Johnson employs a direct and empathetic tone when addressing the nation in this example, thereby establishing a personal and inclusive connection. By using the first person pronoun 'I', he signals a personal connection that conveys responsibility and empathy, indicating to the public that he is personally engaged with their struggles and worries. This notion is further reinforced by the use of the pronoun 'your', thereby making the message feel even more immediate and evoking the impression of a dialogue. The use of parallelism presents the individual grievances as equal and grave, reinforcing the feeling of understanding and empathy. His language appears emotional, with words like 'hard', 'stressful', 'ancient' and 'basic freedoms' evoking strong emotions connected to the loss of traditional rights, thereby highlighting the severity of the restrictions and their massive impact on personal freedoms. This is further emphasised by the negation of terms relating to freedom and normality, such as meeting friends or family. The new reality, characterised by restrictions and isolation, is described next, referencing examples of remote working, juggling childcare, job concerns and company worries. In this part, the focus shifts from personal challenges to the economic ramifications of the crisis, which

---

11 This press statement completely avoids the use of punctuation in the original.

illustrates the prime minister's broader concerns beyond individual discomfort. This example is illustrative of Johnson's use of understanding in his press statements as it demonstrates his recognition of the challenges confronting the public and the business sector, thereby validating the audience's sentiments and experiences. His communication strategy effectively establishes a dialogue-like interaction with the audience that aims to display empathetic understanding, thus providing reassurance and support. This approach not only demonstrates empathy but also fosters a sense of solidarity and patience among the public and business community. Employing a personalised and inclusive method of address, it portrays the prime minister as an involved and caring politician, enabling him to successfully build rapport and create trust, which are essential elements in maintaining public morale and cooperation during challenging times. "Beyond compliance with short-term restrictions, trust is likely to play a key role in citizens' support for/opposition to various other measures as countries work their way out of the pandemic" (Davies et al. 2021: 7). Nevertheless, Johnson often supplements his expressions of understanding with justifications for the necessity of new measures, understanding how crucial gaining public trust is for the crisis situation. The challenging limitations are then portrayed as a crucial sacrifice indispensable for countering the ongoing danger posed by the virus.

In contrast to merely acknowledging these feelings, the next, albeit smaller element in this subcategory, '**sympathising**', also includes sharing a sentiment. The contrast becomes clear in the prime minister's statement from 27 April: "I understand your impatience[.] I share your anxiety" (Johnson 2020l: 2). Whereas the first sentence merely expresses understanding, the second shows that Johnson himself is feeling the same. Another example of this distinction appears in the following comment from a May speech: "I fully acknowledge the difficulties on testing and PPE that we have faced since the start of the outbreak. It has been immensely frustrating, but we are now making progress" (Johnson 2020s: 2). After initially indicating his understanding of the difficult situation, he expresses sympathetic feelings for the frustrated citizens. Nevertheless, in both cases, no change of the existing process has been proposed; instead, he reports a gradual progression on the matter and emphasises the need for caution, citing the potentially catastrophic ramifications of any modification to the government's plan. This further exemplifies the combination of sympathy and subsequent defence of the controversial measure. A total of 27 instances of sympathy were identified in the dataset, primarily expressing concern about the progression of the crisis and its implications for individuals, for example the impact on parenting roles or on businesses. His empathy for citizens' frustrations amid the lengthy restrictions demonstrates an effort to establish an emotional connection with the audience, thereby acknowledging their challenges and validating their feelings. By refraining from proposing immediate changes, his apparent goal is to maintain stability and continuity. This approach may also be intended to circumvent the criticism and confusion that could arise from numerous abrupt shifts in policy. Furthermore, citing potential adverse consequences serves to justify the current course of action, despite negative reactions, and to underscore the gravity of the situation. In conclusion, this speech act appears to be utilised with the intention of reassuring the public, while simultaneously managing their expectations, and maintaining a perception of control during periods of uncertainty.

The third element of the subcategory 'understanding/sympathy' is 'expressing **regret**', which appears 11 times. All of these instances are in the context of Boris Johnson showing regret over the measures his government has declared and the impact they are having on citizens' lives. They occur between the end of March and the beginning of November. Similar to speech acts conveying sympathy, in subsequent sentences Johnson usually asserts that the regulations are inevitable, a necessary consequence of the prevailing circumstances and statistics. The prime minister also displays his emotional struggle through phrases like: "No Prime Minister wants to enact measures like this" (Johnson 2020i: 2). However, expressing regret does not entail a commitment to act differently in the future but rather indicates a desire for a different outcome or a different situation from the outset. His use of speech acts indicating regret therefore seems more like another form of explanation rather than the communication of remorse. It illustrates his conviction that he is acting in the nation's best interest while simultaneously acknowledging the challenges citizens face due to these actions. This subcategory makes up 15% of expressive speech acts.

The final element of this subcategory comprises apologising speech acts. In line with Marsen and Ali-Chand's findings in their 2020 study (cf. 2022: 8), the five instances of **apologies** in the *JPanC20* appear to be inconsequential. It seems that these expressions of regret are not genuine as they are not followed by an assertion of a future change in behaviour. Rather, they represent an attempt to acknowledge the difficulties being experienced by those involved in the situation. This is exemplified by the statement from 31 October: "I am under no illusions about how difficult this will be for businesses which have already had to endure hardship this year. I am truly, truly sorry for that" (Johnson 2020ak: 3). This interpretation of Johnson's apologies in the corpus is reinforced by the fact that the utterances that immediately follow are usually a reaffirmation of the policy for which he has just apologised, e.g.: "I'm afraid it is unavoidable, given the nature of the invisible enemy we are fighting" (Johnson 2020s: 4). Describing it as "unavoidable", the prime minister characterises the situation as one in which the challenging circumstances leave no alternative but to implement the policy in question. This might be an attempt to ensure continued support for the policy by portraying it as a necessity and beyond the leader's control, thus mitigating any negative impact of the apology on his leadership or the policy's acceptance. Consequently, the five cases of apologies do not warrant the establishment of separate subcategory; rather, they have been incorporated into the existing larger subcategory of 'sympathy'.

5.4.1.3 Pride

The next subcategory, titled 'expressing pride', comprises 64 cases. It includes the speech acts 'boast/express pride', 'praise others' and, lastly, 'praise himself/government'. Their distribution within the subcategory is illustrated in figure 6.

Figure 6: Speech act distribution within the subcategory 'pride' in the JPanC20

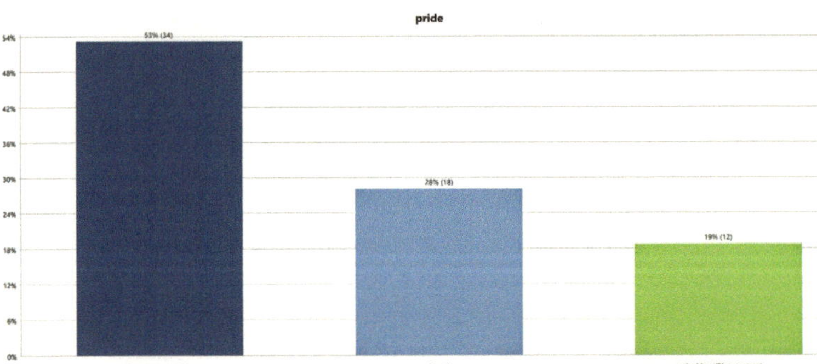

The most frequent speech act in this subcategory is '**boast/express pride**', with 34 instances. Its frequency is not surprising, given that Boris Johnson is expected to show his satisfaction with the government and the nation in his capacity as prime minister. He employs these speech acts frequently throughout the dataset, even at the beginning of the first wave when only limited information about the new virus was available. At the beginning of March, two days before the first British COVID-19 death on 5 March, he boasts: "Let's not forget – we already have a fantastic NHS, fantastic testing systems and fantastic surveillance of the spread of disease" (Johnson 2020a: 1). The repetition of the adjective 'fantastic' emphasises Johnson's confidence in the quality of Great Britain's infrastructure for monitoring and combating this virus, while simultaneously reassuring nervous citizens that the government is well prepared. Although soon confronted with rather disillusioning figures, he continues to express pride in the medical system and the scientific management of the situation. This rhetorical strategy intends to instil confidence in the government's capabilities, even amid growing uncertainty. The expression of pride, particularly in national institutions like the NHS – whose relevance to national identity had already worked as a strong argument during the Brexit debate (cf. Burki 2018: 15f.) – serves to unite the audience around a common identity and bolster collective morale with signs of progress, which is essential for maintaining public cooperation and patience during the unfolding crisis.

Over the following months, Johnson expresses his pride regarding different forms of success in the British response to COVID-19. These include smaller goals, such as the gradual expansion of testing capacities or a variety of inventions by British companies, but also encompass significant events like the completion of the Nightingale Hospitals[12] or the success of vaccine manufacturing. In November and December, he frequently emphasises the successful British vaccine production and the aid programmes that the government delivered during the year. By showcasing these achievements, Johnson conveys a sense of steady progress and active government, thus motivating the public. At the end of the first wave, in July, he summarises the successes of recent months and states proudly:

> "It's vital to stress that we are in a far better position to keep the virus under control now than we were at the start of the pandemic because we know so much more about the virus and have so many more tools at our disposal to deal with it. Our testing capacity has increased 100-fold. We have a contact tracing system up and running which has led to over 184,000 people isolating who may otherwise have spread the virus and is capable of tracing thou-

12 The term 'Nightingale hospital' refers to temporary critical care units within the NHS system, which were established during the COVID-19 pandemic (cf. Proudfoot et al. 2021: 349).

> sands of contacts every day. We have secured supplies of billions of items of PPE to withstand new demands on hospitals and care homes. And of course we have new treatments, like dexamethasone and remdesivir, to shorten recovery times and reduce mortality rates." (Johnson 2020aa: 1)

In this speech, he presents a straightforward list of achievements illustrating the organisational, scientific, technical and medical progress that his government has overseen. He refrains from excessive self-promotion, using the pronoun 'we' and thus allowing the audience to draw their own favourable conclusions. By highlighting specific, measurable successes, Johnson underscores the palpable outcomes of the government's efforts, promoting a narrative of government competence.

In addition to these displays of pride regarding achievements, there are also 18 instances of explicitly **praising others**. These represent the second type of speech act within the subcategory 'pride'. They occur predominantly in May and June, with eight and four instances respectively, i.e. during the period when the first wave of infections is subsiding and restrictions are gradually being relaxed (cf. Knock et al. 2021: 2). The primary addressee is again the British public. Johnson typically discusses a positive development and then proceeds to make statements such as: "That is not my achievement or the government's achievement – it is your achievement, only possible thanks to your resolve and dedication to our national purpose to overcome this virus" (Johnson 2020s: 3). This form of praise gives credit to the public for the progress made, fostering a sense of collective ownership of the success. By downplaying the role of the government in achieving this progress, Johnson once again presents himself as a dedicated and altruistic politician, focusing on the role of the public in this process. With the repeated use of the noun 'achievement', he explicitly emphasises the significance of this accomplishment and frames it in a positive manner, suggesting a notion of collective effort and tangible progress. Instead of enumerating specific, smaller actions that contribute to the positive situation, such as refraining from socialising with friends, staying at home or keeping a distance from others when outside, he places citizens' individual actions within the greater context of "overcome[ing] the virus" and situates them in a heroic narrative of combating a dangerous enemy. Moreover, the selection of the words 'resolve', 'dedication' and 'national purpose' seems rather formal and solemn, thereby underlining the significance and grandeur of this accomplishment and further motivating citizens to continue their cooperative behaviour.

Among the laudatory remarks concerning the British public in general, there is one outlier in the database. This exception might be because of the nature of this speech, which concerns the prime minister's economic vision for the country and was delivered on 30 June. Focusing on life besides the pandemic, Johnson starts by praising Great Britain in general as a great country full of excellent institutions and talents, which his government intends to make even better by specifically supporting them in the areas where they experience challenges. Positioning the nation within a global comparison, he boasts:

> "We have some of the best and most productive companies in the world (...). We have the world's most brilliant medical minds, the world's best pharmaceutical companies, our doctors and treatments are the best in the world (...). We have umpteen fantastic, globally outstanding universities (...). We have a capital city that was, is and will be in so many ways the capital of the world, theatre, finance, tech, restaurants you name it, London leads the world[.]" (Johnson 2020x: 3)

The use of the anaphoric expression 'we have' highlights the presence of a multitude of exemplary institutions and an exceptionally capable workforce, which are described with superlatives such as 'most brilliant', 'best' and 'globally outstanding'. The use of such laudatory adjectives evokes a sentiment of national pride and confidence in the fact that the country occupies an exceptional status on the global stage. The parallel enumerative structure creates a distinctive flow that reinforces the persuasiveness of the argument and evokes an impression of overwhelming evidence supporting the claim of national superiority. The pronoun 'we' positions the speaker as part of the collective, sharing the pride in the nation's achievements and creating an imaginative unity between the speaker and the audience. The reference to London as a world capital that "was, is and will be" suggests a sense of continuity and ongoing greatness, appealing to both nostalgia and optimism about the future, which also translates to the topic of the speech, i.e. the economy. Focusing on behaviour and circumstances during the pandemic, Johnson then pays tribute to the elements of the government that have demonstrated excellence and commitment during the crisis, particularly the British Armed Forces and the UK Treasury:

> "It is our fantastic UK armed services that have played such a crucial role in this crisis, running the test centres, building the hospitals, transporting peo-

> ple from the Shetlands to the right Covid wards. It was the might of the UK Treasury that set up that furlough scheme – in all corners of the country and sent massive and immediate extra funding to all four parts of the UK[.][sic]" (Johnson 2020x: 6)

In contrast to the usual recipients of his praise – typically the citizens of the United Kingdom – in this speech, Johnson directs his attention to several subgroups, including British businesses, scientists, the armed forces and the Treasury. This approach seems an appropriate course of action in his speech, given that the focus is on the economy and these stakeholders have played a pivotal role in getting the economy back on track during the crisis. By drawing attention to these recent success stories, Johnson attempts to construct a compelling narrative highlighting Great Britain's current strengths and achievements. He places an emphasis on what has gone right and frames the pandemic as an opportunity for improvement. The prime minister's narrative seeks to instil confidence in his government's capacity to successfully manage and overcome potential crises. It aims to unite the public by encouraging them to rally behind a shared vision of national excellence and success. Even though laudatory remarks are common in Johnson's rhetoric, and although he displayed considerable confidence at the outset of the pandemic, his open boasting about Britain's superiority as a nation represents a unique phenomenon within the dataset. It seems likely that he intends to channel feelings of national pride and greatness into a sense of optimism about the country's future economic development.

The third part of the subcategory 'pride' comprises speech acts **praising the government or the speaker** himself. In comparison to the considerable number of occasions where citizens are praised, there are relatively few instances of press statements containing self-praise for Johnson or his government. Only 12 cases could be identified, half of which occur in November when he is highlighting the success of the government's economic aid programmes, such as the furlough scheme (cf. Johnson 2020am: 3). In light of the imminent launch of the vaccination campaign and the country's favourable position as the manufacturer of several vaccines, he follows these speech acts by making promises to remain true to his word and to continue the policies outlined earlier, including the timeline provided. This is presented as evidence of the prime minister's reliability and capability as a politician. Two additional instances of self-praise occur in July and August 2020, i.e. a period with a low incidence of cases with restrictions being relaxed and funding being available for government aid programmes designed to assist those experiencing financial difficulties (cf. Knock et al. 2021: 2). Their combination with cautionary speech acts in postposition, which remind the public of the necessity of continued compliance with health measures, suggests a deliberate effort to minimise self-praise, strictly limiting it to periods of favourable circumstances. The next instance is found in October, shortly before the announcement of the second national lockdown: "obviously I am proud that we have massively increased capacity, we do have the Nightingales, we've got 13,000 more nurses now than last year, we have many more doctors" (Johnson 2020ak: 2). Once more, he presents a list of achievements and figures, combining particulars and generalities, thus demonstrating the progress made by his government and the enhanced readiness of the nation to confront forthcoming challenges. The first-person plural pronoun is used, rather than the singular, which signifies that this self-praise is directed at the whole government, rather than the prime minister himself. The qualifiers in this statement range from a concrete number to the less specific terms 'many' and 'massively', which all indicate an increase in preparedness. They reinforce Johnson's message by emphasising the extent and tangible reality of the improvements that have been made. Their intention seems to be to reassure the public of the government's proactive measures and its preparedness. However, the need for this statement, with a cautious tone underlying the self-praise, indicates an awareness of the ongoing challenges and the need for continued vigilance. As this statement is preceded by a warning of potential new restrictions amid the impending infection surge and followed by an expression of confidence in this approach as well as a reminder of past successes – such as improved treatment options and collaboration with particularly affected regions (cf. Johnson 2020ak: 2) – its intention is evident: to remind the audience of the necessity for continued vigilance. In this context, the connotation of caution increases. Consequently, the self-praise appears more like an instance of bolstering rather than outright celebration. Bolstering is a technique commonly employed to "strengthen the audience's positive feelings toward [the speaker](...) in order to offset the negative feelings" (Benoit 1997: 180). Johnson's use of this technique appears to demonstrate the government's capabilities by referencing its prior successes and improvements, while simultaneously acknowledging the ongoing seriousness of the situation.

5.4.1.4 Confidence

The next subcategory, expressing '**confidence**', appears 45 times and only includes this individual speech act. Usually, Johnson's confidence in the measures and his trust in the scientific basis underpinning these decisions is being stated. These utterances serve as both a personal opinion and a persuasive tool, with the objective of convincing the population of the effectiveness of the implemented rules and measures. For instance, in October 2020, Johnson states: "If everyone follows the rule and self-isolates if you have symptoms, get a positive test, or have come into contact with someone who has the virus, we will suppress the disease" (Johnson 2020ah: 3). Expressing confidence in these seemingly easy actions, Johnson aims to enhance public trust in the government's strategy. This assurance is intended to motivate adherence to the guidelines by framing them as easy, but sufficient for controlling the pandemic. The use of a conditional structure presents a clear, achievable goal that depends on collective action, thereby emphasising the power and responsibility of individual behaviour in the greater public health effort.

Johnson's unwavering portrayal of trust in the nation's ability to overcome the threat posed by the virus is evident throughout the dataset, with repeated mentions of the same sentiment expressed in different words. It can be condensed as follows: "I know we are going to succeed and I know we are going to beat this" (Johnson 2020aa: 3). His optimistic and slightly naïve rhetoric even extends to the idea of a stronger return after the crisis, as he emphasised in an evocative manner in his Economy Speech (cf. Johnson 2020x) as well as in his speech from 10 May: "We will come back from this devilish illness. We will come back to health, and robust health. And though the UK will be changed by this experience, I believe we can be stronger and better than ever before" (Johnson 2020m: 5). These statements illustrate his consistent reiteration of optimistic predictions for the future and the prominent emphasis on a resilient national identity. Confident speech acts typically occur at the end of Johnson's press statements, serving as a summative idea of the speech. This pattern of concluding on a positive note reinforces a hopeful outlook and seeks to leave his audience with a lasting impression of optimism and strength. Only ten instances of confident utterances are found at different positions in his speeches, occurring either before or after the announcement of a change in the current rules. With statements such as "we know this sort of intervention works" (Johnson 2020aa: 2), the prime minister emphasises his trust in the effectiveness and evidence-based nature of the government's actions. This strategic placement of confidence is intended to both strengthen public confidence in the implemented measures and show the policy changes in a positive light.

5.4.1.5 Caution

The subcategory expressing '**caution**' refers solely to this individual speech act. It appears 43 times. Only 13 instances are found in the middle sections of the speeches, while the majority occur in the last quarter. Those are either preceded by a report about the success of earlier measures (cf. Johnson 2020ad: 4) or followed by an appeal to stick to the rules and avoid complacency. Most of these are as direct as this request: "we must keep our discipline, we must be focused and we cannot be complacent" (Johnson 2020aa: 2). This use of cautionary speech acts serves to moderate expectations, while also reminding the public of the continuous necessity of adhering to the applicable restrictions. Frequently, this combination of a cautionary speech act and a reminder to stick to the rules also features the current government slogan. These intend to put the main message into one simple and consistent catchphrase for the public to focus on and use as a guide to modify their behaviour. For England, these slogans were used on government websites, in speeches and on lecterns during press conferences (cf. Walker 2021: 1; Nartowski et al. 2020: 48). In May, Johnson cautions that "progress is conditional, provisional. We must keep reducing the incidence of this disease", followed by the final thoughts of the speech: "we must remember the basics. Wash our hands, keep social distance, isolate if you have symptoms – and get a test. We are beating this thing, but we will beat it all the faster if we stay alert, control the virus and save lives" (Johnson 2020q: 3).[13] The prime minister therefore ends with a warning to the audience to stay vigilant and keep up with the COVID-19 restrictions, a frequent occurrence in the dataset. The use of cautionary speech acts contributes to a conservative approach that advises against becoming overly confident at the first signs of success. The same effect can be observed when Johnson discusses the temporal scope of restrictions. Talking about several tests the government has established in the form of a roadmap for the gradual relaxation of rules, his approach becomes evident: "It is vital that these tests are met before any changes are made, because we must not risk all the hard work and sacrifice of the British people" (Johnson 2020s: 1). Citing the sacrifices necessary for the current level of progress, he advocates for patience and carefully considered next actions and decisions. Even though he usually conveys strong confidence

---

13 This slogan 'stay alert, control the virus and save lives' was predominantly used in the period between late April and mid-July 2020 (cf. Callegari 2023: 92). For an overview of British slogans, see Walker (2021).

in the government's crisis management strategy, he concedes that the pandemic "is a complex problem and we are asking for everyone's patience as we work through it together. We will inevitably not get everything right first time" (Johnson 2020s: 4). In this rare acknowledgement that the government's course is likely to encounter challenges and thus will not always succeed in its initial efforts, the prime minister demonstrates a realistic and responsible approach, with the objective of managing public expectations and fostering a sense of collective cooperation and patience. At the same time, he illustrates his commitment to ensuring prudent, conscientious and transparent government action.

5.4.1.6 Anger

The next smallest subcategory is the expression of **anger**, which encompasses 14 instances of reprimanding or angry speech acts. The majority of these pertain to instances of non-compliance with established procedures or regulations. One example of reprimanding took place in connection with Manchester, which was facing a surge of infections necessitating its recategorisation into the "Very High alert level", which signified severe restrictions for residents and businesses. The mayor declined to approve this resolution, prompting Johnson to express his displeasure with regard to the potentially dramatic consequences for the city's inhabitants. Here, he emphasises the importance of time and expresses his lack of understanding for this decision, stating that each day of indecision results in the loss of more lives (cf. Johnson 2020ah: 2). The prime minister explicitly links rule violations to potential increases in fatalities, employing a rhetoric of deterrence aimed at motivating compliance with public health guidelines. This approach underscores the severe consequences of further hesitation, seeking to instil a sense of urgency and responsibility among the addressees, in this case the mayor and the city council. Nevertheless, in the subsequent sentence, he reiterates his offer of cooperation and assistance, citing the effectiveness of joining forces for the benefit of residents. With this approach, Johnson aims to mitigate feelings of resentment and foster a more cooperative atmosphere. It reassures other officials and the public that the government is acting decisively, not only in a punitive manner but also in a supportive one. This emphasises the government's willingness to work collaboratively for mutual benefit. In another example of expressing anger, Johnson conveys his exasperation at those who transgress the rules: "There is nothing more frustrating for the vast majority, the law-abiding majority that do comply[,] than the sight of a few brazenly defying the rules" (Johnson 2020ad: 3).[14] The prime minister's clear and emotive response to rule violations serves as a strong indication to compliant citizens that he values their adherence to the rules, shares their frustration and is determined to uphold order and fairness through decisively addressing non-compliance. This response reinforces a sense of solidarity and collective responsibility while at the same time acting as a deterrent to future rule-breakers. In both examples, just as in the other instances of anger in this dataset, Johnson makes the implicit assertion that he is speaking on behalf of the majority of Britons. This assertion is accompanied by an urgent and rather harsh appeal for the addressees to alter their current non-compliant conduct or their resistance towards his plans or ideas, which makes Johnson appear authentic and relatable.

5.4.1.7 Hope

The subsequent subcategory, expressing '**hope**', appears on 11 occasions in the *JPanC20*. Almost three quarters of hopeful speech acts occur in November. The prime minister conveys his hope that the incoming vaccines will function as a kind of end date for restrictive measures and economic hardship, liberating citizens from the constraints of the pandemic era. Eight of the 11 expressions of hope are related to science, reflecting Johnson's confidence in science-based approaches to resolving the crisis, such as testing and vaccine development. However, it also reflects the government's helplessness, given that these current measures alone have proven insufficient to end the pandemic. Throughout the entire analysis period, Johnson asserts that the development of effective vaccines is a highly anticipated scientific achievement, particularly in the context of the Christmas season (cf. Johnson 2020z: 4). In September, he articulates his only instance of a hopeful speech act regarding the new tests (cf. Johnson 2020ac: 4). He communicates his hope that this innovative tool will accelerate testing capacity in Britain, thereby reversing the current situation of high infection rates. The prime minister avoids explicitly expressing hope during the majority of the period examined, preferring to focus on tangible achievements and actionable plans. This rare exception in September serves to

14 This strict approach does not extend to personal employees or colleagues of the prime minister himself, though, as the case of his political adviser Dominic Cummings demonstrated (cf. Clarke 2021: 7f.; Rathnayake et al. 2023: 474; Holze 2023: 175f.). Besides one brief mention of this incident defending his former employee (cf. Johnson 2020q: 1), Johnson does not comment on his double-standard in the dataset.

highlight the urgent need for enhanced testing capabilities in order to effectively manage the pandemic, whereas the high number of such statements in November stresses the hope he places in the vaccine campaign to finally lift restrictions for Britons. It may also reflect the considerable pressure that Johnson had been under since the announcement of the second lockdown within eight months.

5.4.1.8 Relief

For the next subcategory, seven instances of expressing **relief** were identified. They comprise comments on positive news delivered in the corresponding press statement, such as a reopening of public places or infection rates going down. One example can be identified in this July statement: "I am pleased to report that we have continued to make steady progress in our collective effort to beat the coronavirus" (Johnson 2020z: 1). All seven instances occurred in the period between May and July, during the decline of the first wave of infections in Great Britain (cf. Knock et al. 2021: 3). The prime minister is therefore expressing his relief that the government's measures, e.g. the first lockdown, have been effective, which reinforces his image as an authentic leader. The timing of these statements suggests that Johnson may have been under great pressure during this initial phase of the pandemic and is relieved that his policies were effective, as evidenced by receding infection rates.

5.4.1.9 Grief

The subcategory 'express **grief**' occurs in only five cases, four of which were in May. In this month, the restrictions of the initial lockdown were gradually being lifted, and the high number of fatalities became apparent (cf. Knock et al. 2021: 2)[15]. Johnson responds to these figures with statements such as "Every day brings heart-breaking news as more lives are lost before their time to this vicious coronavirus. Every victim leaves behind family, friends and loved ones who mourn their loss. They remain constantly in my thoughts" (Johnson 2020p: 1). Through this declaration, Johnson seeks to convey empathy and solidarity

15 At these critical moments, other scholars found instances of blaming and scapegoating from different members of Johnson's government towards scientists and other experts (cf. Pearse 2020: 574) as well as towards the British public (cf. Morgan 2020: 299), "in particular as the easing of restrictions resulted in spikes in infection and death rates" (Lilleker and Stoeckle 2021: 7). These are not detected in this dataset, however.

with the public in this time of collective grief and social isolation. He acknowledges the emotional impact of the situation and demonstrates awareness of the personal toll on families and loved ones. This approach aims to humanise statistical data and reassure citizens that their suffering is recognised at the highest levels of government. His intention might be to reinforce a collective resolve against the virus. However, the rarity of these statements indicates that the prime minister employed them sparingly and mostly in the context of the initial wave of the pandemic. A constant and sorrowful reminder of fatalities could have the effect of highlighting the ineffectiveness and delayed response of the British government. Consequently, the frequent issuing of mourning statements was not a component of his communication strategy.

5.4.1.10 Impatience

The expression of **impatience** occurs just three times within the dataset, which makes it a rather minor subcategory within expressives. While Johnson impatiently acknowledges the difficulties with testing and with obtaining the required protective equipment in May (cf. Johnson 2020s: 2), he employs the metaphor of a nightmare that he is impatient to leave behind to describe the situation in June (cf. Johnson 2020x: 1). Two months later, he joins the ranks of those who admit to feeling fed up with the numerous restrictions (cf. Johnson 2020af: 1). In all these cases, he is signalling his understanding of the public's increasing frustration with the ongoing regulations and measures. His second and third expressions of impatience are followed by an appeal to persevere and continue to adhere to the current rules as "there is only one way of doing this" (Johnson 2020af: 1). In contrast, the first occurrence in the dataset makes the assertion that, after all the frustrating delays, progress is finally being made. Johnson's open displays of impatience convey a sense of authenticity and relatability, as they acknowledge the shared sentiments of fatigue and exasperation among the public. This fosters a connection with his audience while reinforcing the necessity of ongoing compliance, which might motivate them to continue complying.

5.4.1.11 Hedging/deflecting

The subcategory '**hedging/deflecting**' appears relatively infrequently, with these speech acts occurring only ten times within this dataset. The British prime minister employs a small range of cautious language to express his hesitation about providing definite numbers or to indicate that the information on future action he has just provided is subject to change, depending on evolving circumstances and scientific recommendations (see also Holze 2023: 184). One statement illustrating this approach reads as follows: "today [there is] a general consensus on what we could do. And I stress could. Because although we have a plan, it is a conditional plan" (Johnson 2020m: 2). Johnson's emphasis of the conditional 'could' implies a cautious and provisional stance, indicating that while there is agreement on potential actions within the government, these are not definite or guaranteed. He stresses the limitations of the presented provisional roadmap, which is contingent on the availability of new information or scientific advice, in the context of the evolving conditions surrounding the crisis. Employing this rhetorical device allows the prime minister flexibility in navigating the unpredictable nature of the pandemic while still conveying an optimistic and confident outlook. Thus, the use of hedging enables the government to manage the public's expectations and avoid overcommitting to specific outcomes or timelines that may prove undeliverable, given the dynamic and unpredictable nature of the circumstances.

5.4.1.12 Personal experience

Only four utterances have been found in which Boris Johnson talks about his **personal experience** with COVID-19. The earliest is from the end of March, when he informs the public of his positive test result and mild symptoms. He uses this experience as a positive example for others, emphasising his status as a self-isolating remote worker. He further asserts that this course of action is "entirely the right thing to do" (Johnson 2020k: 1). By positioning himself as a role model for other patients, he hopes to encourage other infected Britons to follow his lead. The prime minister ends this announcement paragraph with the reassurance that he is doing relatively well and is positive about being able to continue working. Continuing with praise for modern technology, medical staff and other keyworkers, he stresses his gratefulness and his conviction that the nation will get through what was then an epidemic. He concludes this relatively brief statement with a request for the public to follow his example and comply with official measures. Johnson is therefore using his own infection to model desired behaviour and stress the importance of following the rules.

Two more instances of talking about his personal experience took place at the press conference on 27 April 2020, after he had been infected and had been seriously ill for several weeks (cf. The Guardian 2020). He said: "If this virus were a physical assailant[,] an unexpected and invisible mugger[,] which I can tell you from personal experience it is[,] then this is the moment when we have begun together to wrestle it to the floor" (Johnson 2020l: 1). Here, the prime minister uses his personal experience as an intensifier to add weight and credibility to his message. The use of vivid imagery, such as comparing the virus to an invisible mugger, makes his message more memorable and powerful. It provides a visual representation of the threat to hitherto unexposed members of the public and emphasises the necessity for collective action to overcome it. Furthermore, disclosing his struggle makes him appear more approachable and evokes a feeling of empathy among those who have also been impacted by the virus. Linking the illness to an inconspicuous passer-by serves to emphasise the unexpected nature of the infection and its potential to affect anyone. In contrast to his social media videos and interviews from this time, Johnson rarely discusses his personal experience of the virus at official press conferences. One reason for this might be that a persistent focus on the subject of his illness could give rise to queries regarding his present state of health and fitness for the role of prime minister, potentially generating unwarranted distractions or concerns about his ability to govern the country (cf. McGuire et al. 2020: 365). The last time he mentions his personal experience in the dataset is in his speech to the United Nations General Assembly in September, where he maximises his credibility and the impact of his words by emphasising that he is speaking "as a former COVID patient" (Johnson 2020ae: 1). These four mentions account for only 1% of the expressive speech acts.

5.4.1.13 Expressive speech acts – summary

In conclusion, the prevalence of expressive speech acts, which make up a third of all speech acts in this dataset, indicates that they constitute a significant aspect of Johnson's communicative style. He employs them regularly to illustrate his authenticity, render his decisions more relatable or persuade citizens to adhere to his directives or new restrictions. The prime minister's statements are characterised by a notable prevalence of expressions of gratitude, praise and confidence, with positive emotions accounting for nearly 60% of the 424 expressive speech acts. His frequent acknowledgement of and gratitude towards others indicate a strategy of recognising and appreciating the contributions of various groups for their role in mitigating the crisis, for example healthcare workers, essential personnel and the general public. This positive reinforcement encourages and validates their efforts, demonstrating that everyone's contribution is impactful and valued by the government and their community, which reinforces a sense of unity and shared responsibility. It is a common practice in Johnson's crisis communication to highlight both minor and major successes and achievements, thus reassuring the public that their efforts are yielding positive results. By emphasising the importance of incremental progress, Johnson communicates a message of persistence and resilience, indicating that the nation is on the right track even if the pace of advancement is not as fast as desired. This approach also mitigates the risk of public disillusionment, as it sets realistic expectations and underscores the notion that consistent effort, rather than dramatic or immediate actions, will ultimately lead to success. He often combines this with praise for different subgroups or the public as a whole, situating individual actions within a greater heroic narrative of combating a vicious enemy. This contributes to a feeling of urgency and collective ownership of successes. One frequent recipient of his appreciation is the National Health Service (NHS), which already points to the government's priority of avoiding an overwhelmed medical system.

One essential objective of his communication strategy seems to be to create a positive outlook. By focusing on positive emotions, this strategy can help to alleviate fear and anxiety among the public, emotions which are likely to be prevalent during a pandemic. During periods of crisis, individuals tend to seek guidance and confidence from their leaders (cf. Liu et al. 2020: 128). The prime minister articulates his unwavering confidence in the efficacy of the measures and strategies implemented by his administration, thus instilling a sense of confidence and stability while also fulfilling the public's need for reassurance. Where he cannot give a timeline or commit to specific actions, he sometimes employs hedging to manage public expectations. By emphasising gratitude, praise and confidence, Johnson seeks to provide a counterbalance to the frustration, isolation and stress caused by the crisis, which is essential for fostering compliance and resilience among citizens. The frequency of speech acts that demonstrate understanding and sympathy, amounting to 21% of the expressive speech acts, contributes to this approach by creating an empathic connection between the prime minister and the public. This signals to citizens that the government is aware of the sacrifices it is demanding from its constituents and is not announcing new measures arbitrarily, which enhances trust and ongoing cooperation. Furthermore, demonstrating an understanding of the difficulties faced by the general public can reinforce the perception of authenticity, a central element of Johnson's rhetoric, and illustrate his relatable nature to the general population. This, in turn, serves to bolster public morale and foster a sense of solidarity during the crisis.

Negative or hesitant emotions, mainly expressions of caution, which account for around 10% of expressive speech acts, are less frequent in the dataset. Cautionary statements call for adherence to the rules and the avoidance of complacency. They tend to advise against overconfidence after reports of success and are often made in times of rising infection rates. Anger is common on the rare occasions when violations of the rules are discussed, or when offers of cooperation are rejected despite warnings. Johnson presents such cases as an insult to those working hard to comply with the rules and as a threat to the collective commitment needed to combat the virus. Nevertheless, as anger and impatience combined represent less than 5% of expressive speech acts within this corpus, it seems that the prime minister tends to maintain self-control in public and rarely exhibits anger. Grief is even less apparent, suggesting a general emphasis on maintaining a composed and resilient demeanour. The expressions of regret or apology in the dataset seem to function more as explanations with a reaffirmation of policy rather than as communications of remorse. Instead of pledging to do things differently in the future, Johnson tends to emphasise his belief that the measures were necessary, despite being inconvenient and challenging. The aim is to persuade the audience to follow the rules, however difficult that may be. It also portrays the government as almost infallible, which appears in line with his often-stated confidence in his government's strategy and policies.

Johnson rarely refers to his personal experience as a COVID-19 patient, potentially to avoid any questioning of his leadership skills. When he does, he uses it to model the desired behaviour of an infected person and to stress the importance of following the rules. The essence of his statements concerning his personal experience, in combination with understanding speech acts and those expressing frustration or grief, seems to be a call to the nation to abide by the rules, however frustrating and difficult that may be. In addition, these emotions portray the prime minister as an ordinary individual facing challenges similar to those of the general public, including the experience of isolation and the limitations imposed by the situation. This supports his communication strategy by humanising his leadership, demonstrating empathy and reinforcing the need for collective compliance with public health measures. By sharing his own challenges and expressing shared emotions, he aims to build trust, foster solidarity and motivate the public to continue complying despite the hardships.

Expressive speech acts thus fulfil two distinct functions: firstly, they intend to reinforce the nation's confidence in the government and its implemented measures, and secondly, they emphasise the ongoing necessity for the public to adhere to the current restrictions.

5.4.2 Assertive speech acts

A total of 364 occurrences of assertives have been identified, encompassing on average 363 characters with spaces included, which is almost a quarter of the respective press statement (cf. Johnson 2020y: 2f.). The longest assertive expression contains 2,210 characters, whereas the shortest has only 30 (cf. figure A5).

Assertives are divided into the seven subcategories 'explain', 'report', 'affirm', 'state', 'narrate', 'describe' and 'answer'. Figure 7 gives an overview of the distribution of assertive speech acts in the *JPanC20*.

Figure 7: Subcategory percentages within the category 'Assertives' in the JPanC20

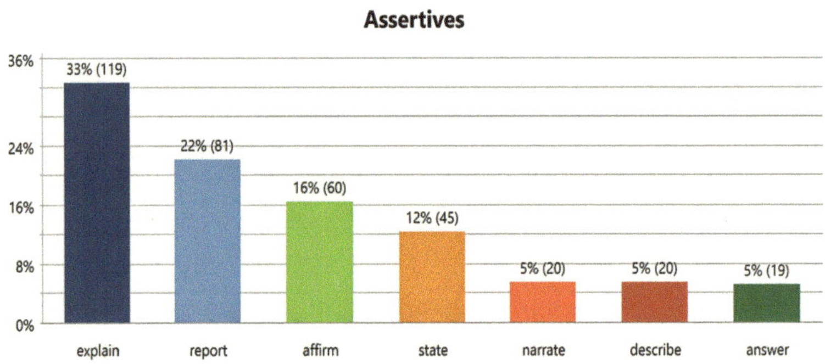

5.4.2.1 Explain

The subcategory '**explain**' is the most frequent, with 119 instances accounting for 33% of assertive utterances. This speech act encompasses three distinct areas of explanation: the ongoing danger posed by the virus, the rationale behind the proposed measures and the impact of these measures on the crisis.

One focus of Johnson's communication is explaining the virus's mechanisms and the statistical data on which the government's policies are based. Most frequently explained are the reasons for and the measures associated with lockdowns, mentioned on 13 occasions, as well as information about the virus itself, such as the mechanisms of transmission, with 14 occurrences. As these are the topics that arose first chronologically and caused the country to change everyday personal and communal habits in a dramatic way, Johnson might have felt that they needed more explanation than others. Additionally, during the first lockdown, which includes a significant part of this dataset, these two issues were among the most pressing matters in need of clarification. However, as the situation evolved, a multitude of new challenges emerged, necessitating explanations on a range of subjects, such as tests, vaccines or the rules for the Christmas holidays. Furthermore, given the unprecedented nature of a situation characterised by uncertainty and a sense of apprehension, the public sought guidance and information as they were unable to develop an informed opinion independently. Similarly, there are ten instances where the meaning of the presented numbers is elaborated upon, along with their consequences for citizens, such as rising infection rates in autumn, which could signify an impending winter surge. Explaining the circumstances and implications of the figures presented at the beginning of most press conferences is therefore an important part of Johnson's communication strategy throughout the dataset.

Prior to or following the declaration of novel regulations, Boris Johnson presents the reasons why they are necessary and the rationale behind the government's decision. One example is the press statement from 31 October, where he provides a comprehensive account of the necessity of the planned November lockdown:

> "And let me explain why the overrunning of the NHS would be a medical and moral disaster beyond the raw loss of life. Because the huge exponential growth in the number of patients to treat[,] Who would get oxygen and who wouldn't[,] Who would live and who would die, And doctors and nurses would be forced to choose between saving covid patients and non-covid patients[,] And the sheer weight of covid demand would mean depriving tens of thousands, if not hundreds of thousands, if not millions, of non-covid patients of the care they need[,][sic]" (Johnson 2020ak: 2)

The prime minister attempts to explain the reason for the imposition of a new lockdown in a clear and accessible manner. By employing a deliberate and straightforward style of communication, he aims to facilitate comprehension among the general public and encourage their support for the measures, despite the potential personal challenges and implications. With regard to the medical situation at that time, he provides a detailed account of the probable consequences and their extent, intending to enable citizens without a medical or scientific background to understand the considerations behind this decision. Thus, Johnson attempts to foster acceptance of his measures by using explanatory speech acts that elucidate their intended effects. The NHS is once again employed as a point of reference. Firstly, this is due to the necessity of providing medical care for individuals affected by COVID-19, despite the already considerable pressure on healthcare resources. Secondly, it is regarded as a national institution that is held in high esteem by the majority of citizens, who want to see it preserved.

The ramifications of new regulations for schools were explained on eight occasions. As the government declared it a priority to maintain the presence of children in educational institutions (cf. Johnson 2020q: 2), the specifics were conveyed explicitly to provide guidance and reassurance to parents, educators and administrative bodies. During the second half of the year, the public's attention shifted towards funding plans as well as to local or regional measures. Both issues are mentioned on eight occasions in the context of an explanation by the prime minister. However, the government's answer to the problem of businesses being unable to sustainably pay their workers due to reduced income during the lockdown period was presented by the then-Minister of Finance, Rishi Sunak, instead of the prime minister, who only refers to Sunak's statements on this. Boris Johnson thus often employs his press statements as a platform to clarify operational procedures and to reassure both workers and businesses that they will be supported, though he does not announce these particular policies himself.

This approach of providing easily understandable explanations and focusing on the well-being of citizens is also evident in his remarks regarding local and regional measures. One notable example is the introduction of a system of regional alert levels with four tiers, which are explained on nine occasions in the period from October to December. A new feature on the government website, which allows for straightforward verification of the active level in each region of England, prompts this explanation: "You will shortly be able to type in your postcode into Gov.UK and see exactly what restrictions apply where you live. The majority of the country will, for now, be at medium. Most areas currently under local intervention will be at High[sic]" (Johnson 2020ag: 2). Here, he presents a clear and user-oriented explanation of the new tool's functionality in easy terms for the public, while also outlining the anticipated outcomes, which serves to allay fears surrounding the unfamiliar technology. Besides this new feature, Johnson addresses other pertinent issues, including the various regulations beyond the lockdown and regional measures (six mentions), the NHS strategy (six), the test and trace system (six) and details regarding the different vaccines in development (four). In summary, the introduction of new measures that affect the entire population, including lockdowns, the 'Rule of 6' and the specifics of handwashing prompt the prime minister to provide frequent explanations, as they are the new guidelines for community life in England. More specific rules, e.g. the new border laws, are addressed significantly less often.

The assertive speech act 'explain' therefore embodies the informative and instructive function of crisis communication (cf. Olsson and Eriksson 2020: 420), providing clarity and transparency about the new measures and the behaviours expected from Britons. Concurrently, the communication of the underlying thought process and figures on which the new restrictions are based enables the prime minister to inform the public and encourage compliance through understanding, with the ultimate objective of cultivating a sense of collective responsibility. To a lesser extent, this speech act also fulfils the strategic component described by Marsen and Ali-Chand (2022: 8) by asserting authority and leading the discourse.

5.4.2.2 Report

The second subcategory of assertives, **'report'**, can be found 81 times. It encompasses the three elements 'report' (43 instances), 'update' (23) and 'give examples' (15). An overview of their distribution is provided in figure 8.

Figure 8: Speech act distribution within the subcategory 'report' in the JPanC20

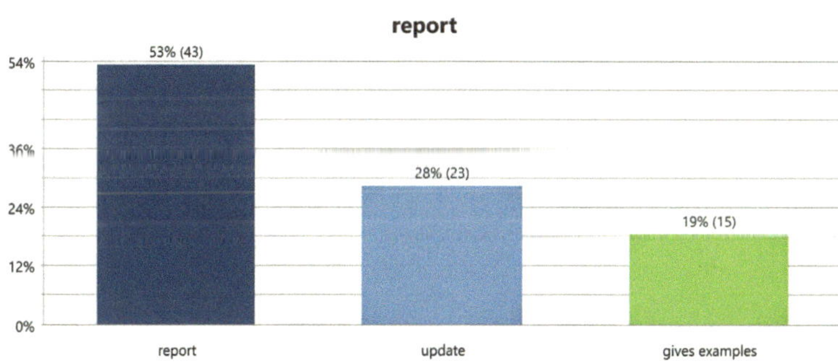

The first of these elements, **reporting** speech acts, frequently includes progress announcements regarding predefined performance indicators, referred to as the 'five tests', which serve as a benchmark to determine whether more stringent measures are necessary (cf. Johnson 2020v: 1f.). These often utilise precise numerical data, specified for all parts of the United Kingdom. The following example illustrates this speech act: "On 7 June, 443 people were admitted to hospital with coronavirus in England, Wales and Northern Ireland, down from 628 two weeks earlier, and down from a peak of 3,431 on 1 April" (Johnson 2020v: 1). Additionally, the prime minister uses spatial and temporal deixis, in particular when in reporting whether the 'five tests' have been satisfied: "[we have] procured 2.2 billion items of PPE to be manufactured domestically. Despite the immensely frustrating difficulties we have faced with PPE and testing in the past, this progress means we are now satisfied that the fourth test is being met" (Johnson 2020v: 2). The deictic expressions, such as 'domestically' and 'now' in this example, anchor his assessments firmly within the context of Great Britain, as articulated by a British national to a British audience.

Additionally, information about planned or concluded events is summarised within this category, for example: "Tomorrow, there will be a moment of remembrance for those whose lives have tragically been lost before their time" (Johnson 2020y: 3). The actual information provided regarding the planned event is presented in a relatively neutral and informative manner, with the introduction of more emotive language only in reference to the individuals at the centre of the said event. Johnson's reporting speech acts therefore contribute to the informative function of crisis communication, with the objective of providing information in context for the public.

The second element of 'report', '**updates**', typically encompass an overview of new figures, which include a variety of details on the R-rate[16], infection or death numbers, testing numbers and hospitalisation rates. In some instances, these updating speech acts are accompanied by a slideshow during the press conference (cf. Allen et al. 2024), which is in some cases mentioned verbally but is excluded from the current analysis since the slideshow is not accessible via the government website. In these cases, he explains the graphs depicted in the accompanying slide and reports the latest developments in the field by mentioning the exact figures and contextualising them. This results in a high co-occurrence of this speech act and the aforementioned speech act of 'explaining'. Except for five cases out of the 23 updates in the dataset, all are located in

16 'R-rate', or more briefly, 'R', refers to the reproduction rate of the virus. It is one of the key statistic figures in the British communication on the pandemic.

the initial section of the press statement, as the prime minister frequently begins his speech by presenting the latest figures required in the so-called 'five tests'. One typical example is the following statement from 24 May:

> "So let me give you today's figures: 3,458,905 tests for coronavirus have now been carried out in the UK, including 110,401 tests carried out yesterday. 259,559 people have tested positive, that's an increase of 2,409 cases since yesterday – a smaller increase than we were seeing over the last few weeks. 8,951 people are in hospital with COVID-19 in the UK, down 11% from 10,085 this time last week. And sadly, of those tested positive for coronavirus, across all settings, 36,793 have now died. That's an increase of 118 fatalities since yesterday." (Johnson 2020q: 1)

Here, the prime minister employs a simple and matter-of-fact style of language, refraining from emotional commentary or broader contextualisation of the presented data besides brief one-word comments expressing grief, such as 'sadly' or 'tragically'. While 'sadly' occurs six times across all updating speech acts, always before the current number of new deaths is disclosed, 'tragic*' occurs only once; this takes place on 30 September, when reporting a significant increase in daily deaths (cf. Johnson 2020af: 1). For comparison, the absolute numbers in the dataset are 21 for the lemma 'sad*' and 11 for 'trag*', including one occurrence of its nominalisation 'tragedy'. Following the initial mention of the current number of cases within a given category, Johnson usually provides contextualisation by presenting the percentage or absolute number within a specified timeframe. In response to these updates, he typically reiterates that progress is being made and provides a summary of any positive developments, such as: "while we mourn every death, the average daily death rate continues, steadily, to fall" (Johnson 2020z: 1). Additionally, he often reaffirms the advice provided by his scientific advisory council and sets out his preferred course of action in light of the circumstances. These speech acts are thus intended to inform the public about new developments and contextualise the presented figures.

The third element in the subcategory 'report' – '**giving examples**' – is employed in instances where Johnson explicitly discusses a particular situation in a specific location. This is done to demonstrate his ability to address local issues and his awareness of the nuances of these problems. In all cases where he provides updates, he reports on the effectiveness of the actions taken by his administration in addressing the situation, for example: "In Weston-Super-

Mare, we identified an outbreak in a hospital, closed it to visitors and new admissions, tested all staff and patients and gave the hospital a deep clean. The outbreak was contained and the hospital is open again[sic]" (Johnson 2020y: 2). The statement's action-oriented language, comprising active verbs such as 'identified', 'closed', 'tested' and 'contained', emphasises the proactive measures taken to address the outbreak, with the use of the past tense indicating that the events in question have already come to a conclusion. The verbs are arranged in a sequential order that highlights the systematic and organised steps that were taken, thereby indicating a methodical approach. The efficacy of these measures in containing the outbreak illustrates the effectiveness of the government's response. The subject of the sentence is indicated by the pronoun 'we'. In this context, it indicates a particular subgroup that includes the prime minister himself, rather than the government or the nation as a whole. It can be assumed that this group is made up of a team within the broader community of emergency responders, acting as service providers to the public. Portraying himself as one of them, Johnson is presented as a capable, caring and successful official actively working for the betterment of the people. The tone of the statement is reassuring and aims to instil confidence in the public by conveying that the situation is under control, while the simple and matter-of-fact language helps to convey a message of competence and successful crisis management. Giving examples like the one above therefore acts as an empirical demonstration of the government's capacity, showing its efficacy and proficiency in navigating the pandemic.

5.4.2.3 Affirm

The third subcategory of assertives is **affirm**. It includes 60 assertive speech acts and is subdivided into 'affirming' itself, with 31 instances, and 'affirming prior policies', with 29 instances, as illustrated in figure 9.

Figure 9: Speech act distribution within the subcategory 'affirm' in the JPanC20

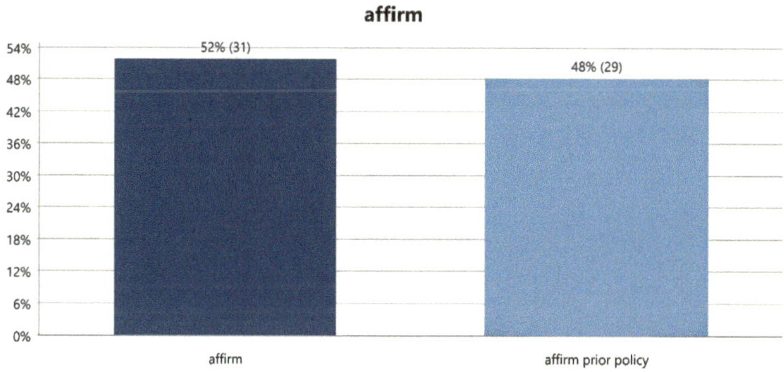

The first element consists of several instances of **affirmation** that the government's chosen priorities are still in place and that it is still meeting its objectives. An example from March 2020 reads: "And that's why keeping the country safe is the government's overriding priority. And our plan means we're committed to doing everything possible based on the advice of our world leading scientific experts to prepare for all eventualities[sic]" (Johnson 2020a: 1). This comment reaffirms the government's commitment to the roadmap that was previously introduced. The introductory phrase "and that's why" effectively links Johnson's statement to the earlier explanation for the measures, pointing to a systematic and thorough approach. This is also reflected in the anaphoric syntax, which creates a logical link and reinforces the argument that the prime minister is acting methodically and deliberately. The term "overriding priority" acknowledges the existence of other important elements in the pandemic, all of which are presented as secondary to the security of the country, thus reassuring the nation of the government's determination to keep them safe. Basing its response on the expertise of "world leading scientific experts" justifies the choice of these policies and enhances the legitimacy of the proposed measures, as this phrase conveys authority and credibility while simultaneously discouraging dissent, for example from the opposition. This is achieved by aligning the government's measures with those set out in internationally accepted scientific literature. Johnson's intention seems to be to reassure the public that the government has everything under control and is being guided by knowledgeable advisers, thus instilling confidence and trust. In response to anticipated concerns from the audience about security, the speaker employs assertive language to address these concerns and provide reassurance, expressing his stance that the government's behaviour is appropriate and proportionate to the situation.

By contrast, the second element of this subcategory, '**affirmation of prior policies**', includes statements insisting that previous policies were correct, even though the figures may not appear successful at the current moment. In some cases, this culminates in a call for the policies to be continued: "But as we've said over the last few weeks, we have a clear plan that we are now working through" (Johnson 2020c: 1), highlighting the government's unwavering dedication to the established plan and asserting its validity and necessity. The reference to the earlier plan, now being implemented, portrays Johnson as an experienced politician undeterred by initial setbacks. Statements like this serve to reinforce the belief that the current course of action remains appropriate, thereby reassuring the public and strengthening confidence in the government's decisions. Both types of affirming speech acts seem to be equally important for the prime minister's strategy. Overall, affirmative speech acts emphasise the stringency of the government's policies and counter complaints from the opposition and the public that they might be too flexible and lack a clear, sustainable plan.

5.4.2.4 State

The fourth subcategory of assertives, '**state**', occurs 45 times. It is solely comprised of this speech act type. In around half of these occurrences, Johnson expresses facts or statements that he considers to be unquestionably true, such as: "The coronavirus is the biggest threat this country has faced for decades – and this country is not alone" (Johnson 2020i: 1). His utterance presents his perspective as factual by using the present tense and builds on the first assertion with the second part of the sentence. By using absolute language, he characterises the pandemic as the most dangerous threat to Britain in decades, thereby constructing a narrative of unparalleled danger that leaves little room for dissent or criticism. In comparing the British situation to that of other countries, an idea found 14 times in the dataset, he implies that the current problems are not the result of the (in-)actions of his government but rather the consequence of the nature of this crisis. This effectively frames the discourse in a way that asserts the unassailability of his position.

Moreover, on 16 occasions, stating speech acts are used for announcements of new projects, measures or proceedings that are in preparation or underway. Utterances such as, "On Monday I will set out our plans to parliament.

On Wednesday, parliament will debate and vote on these measures which, if passed, will (...) come into force on Thursday" (Johnson 2020ak: 3), serve a preparatory function. The rather brief, anaphoric sentences help to orient the audience in advance of what is to come. In this instance, the objective is to provide a definitive timeline for the implementation of the proposed measures, thereby ensuring a clear understanding of the anticipated timeframe and managing public expectations.

In addition to these absolute statements and announcements, Johnson reiterates his assertions from the preceding days or weeks on 12 occasions. These emphasise the coherence of his policies and his dedication to the objectives and schedules set out earlier. The following comment is an example of this: "Two weeks ago, I (...) said that from tomorrow the government would give employers more discretion over how employees can work safely" (Johnson 2020aa: 2). It is followed by a reaffirmation of the established guidelines, citing the necessity for sustained vigilance and discipline as reasons for not loosening the strict rules at workplaces, as well as praising those employers who have demonstrated compliance with the aforementioned recommendations. The prime minister's reiteration of his earlier commitment, presented in the past tense, is complemented by the use of simple vocabulary, which facilitates comprehension for all citizens. Maintaining the scheduled timeline for this update conveys reliability and a coherent plan of action.

5.4.2.5 Describe

The three minor subcategories of assertive speech acts – '**describe**', 'narrate' and 'answer' – each account for 5% of the dataset. Descriptions, occurring 20 times in the analysed period, encompass Johnson's detailed accounts of a situation or set of circumstances pertaining to a given measure. Primarily, he describes the circumstances and working of his measures (13 occurrences) and medical procedures (four occurrences), such as the methodology behind saliva tests for COVID-19 detection (cf. Johnson 2020ac: 4). He tries to make the procedures more understandable and relatable for the audience by employing straightforward and simple language, while avoiding excessive medical terminology. In some cases, he also outlines the possible new reality resulting from the planned measures, e.g. when describing the effects of saliva tests:

> "That level of testing would allow people to lead more normal lives, without the need for social distancing: Theatres and sports venues could test all audience members on the day and let in those with a negative result, all those

> who are not infectious. Workplaces could be opened up to all those who test negative that morning and allow them to behave in a way that was normal before COVID." (Johnson 2020ac: 4)

Here, Johnson outlines a potential new normality that incorporates cherished elements of everyday life from before the pandemic – things that had been impossible for some months – such as watching theatre plays or going to sports matches with larger audiences. He also mentions the potential for returning to the workplace in person, rather than continuing to work from home. These examples provide the public with a number of concrete scenarios, enabling a deeper understanding of the potential benefits and applications of this innovative technology while highlighting the significant advancements it might represent for them personally. The selection of these three particular activities, namely watching a play, engaging in sports and going to work, is intended to appeal to a broad range of Britons, as their interests are likely to involve at least one of these activities. Moreover, he differentiates between two groups: those who have tested negative and are therefore not infectious – and can thus resume all normal activities – and those who do not meet these criteria and must continue to maintain physical distance. By presenting several optimistic scenarios, Johnson motivates the audience and encourages them to consider the opportunities that would be feasible should this new kind of test be successfully deployed nationwide. However, he still presents these in a cautious manner by using the modal verbs 'would' and 'could' to describe a hypothetical reality, thereby portraying himself as a politician who weighs his actions and decisions carefully.

Johnson gives a description of the global or local situation four times. Despite acknowledging unfavourable developments, he attempts to deflect responsibility from his government and instead attribute it to the inherent characteristics of the pandemic. He contextualises the crisis in a manner that fosters a sense of collective experience and empathy within the nation in light of comparable developments in other countries within Europe (cf. Johnson 2020ak: 1f.). As with the subcategory 'state', describing speech acts do not invite criticism or dissent from the presented interpretation, which the prime minister portrays as factual.

5.4.2.6 Narrate

The subcategory '**narrate**' occurs 20 times and is used to convey a situation or experience in a particularly poetic way. Johnson's usual diction is already known for "linguistic originality" (Charteris-Black 2019: 168) as well as his "highly diverse inventory of rhetorical and stylistic devices" (Abramicheva 2022: 4; see also Heaney and Riboni 2023), in particular the frequent use of metaphors that "break the normal conventions of language and delight in imaginative fantasy" (Charteris-Black 2019: 168). Similarly, his rhetoric in the dataset appears to be particularly poetic in certain instances. A substantial proportion (60%) of these narrating speech acts are located in the initial section of the press statement, thereby establishing the tone for the subsequent presentation of new information. Although this subcategory mainly occurs in November (60%), when it is employed to highlight the substantial and ongoing risks as well as the promise of incoming vaccines, Johnson deploys this device most frequently in his address to the UN General Assembly. Here, he applies this speech act four times, one of which is this utterance: "Never in the history of our species – not since the Almighty felled the Tower of Babel – has the human race been so obsessed with one single topic of conversation" (Johnson 2020ae: 1). In this example, he is emphasising the common ground between people of all nations by addressing their identity as a species and "human race". Johnson draws a parallel between a religious narrative of an epic event, which can be found in numerous religious traditions, and the present circumstances in order to underscore the global impact of the pandemic. As with the aforementioned example of the speech act 'state', his presentation of the events highlights the pandemic as a significant international caesura. By making this interpretation of the situation more prominent through his extraordinary and poetic language, he attempts to persuade the attending delegations to act beyond the scope of their usual policy strategies. An additional comment at the occasion reinforces this interpretation by emphasising the divisive impact of the virus on a global scale. Here, the urgent need for a unified approach to combating the virus is referred to again with regard to vaccines, which are needed everywhere regardless of borders (cf. Johnson 2020ae: 2f.). In this subcategory, he employs a highly figurative and elaborate rhetorical style to illustrate his perspective on the situation in a vivid and descriptive manner. With this method, he engages the delegates' imagination and emotions, thereby enhancing the impact and relatable nature of the message. By crafting a compelling narrative, he can subtly influence the audience's perception and align it with his perspective of thinking beyond national borders. Besides employing the religious trope of the Tower of Babel in a narrating speech act, Johnson also borrows metaphoric images from mythology, such as referencing the Greek monsters Scylla and Charybdis on 22 October, or the Cloak of Invisibility on 19 March, which may reference a Welsh myth about King Arthur's cloak (cf. Finke and Shichtman 2007: 101). However, especially among younger members of the audience, it might be more closely associated with the *Harry Potter* series, where such a cloak plays an essential role (cf. Rowling 1999: 201). These cultural references evoke narratives that are widely recognised and understood, facilitating the effective communication of complex ideas and enhancing the memorability of his speeches.

The other occurrences of narrating speech acts mostly highlight the progress that has been achieved (eight instances) or illustrate the dangerous nature of the virus itself (six instances). The following statement represents one example of the first phenomenon: "The breakthroughs in treatment, in testing and vaccines mean that the scientific cavalry is now in sight and we know in our hearts that next year we will succeed" (Johnson 2020aq: 1).[17] This vivid metaphor suggests that breakthroughs in different research areas will be instrumental in delivering victory over the pandemic. Moreover, he indicates that this state will become a reality in the near future and provides a concrete temporal anchor for the resolution of the crisis. Establishing a connection to the WAR frame, it portrays science as a heroic saviour figure coming to the rescue of the nation, thereby reinforcing a sense of hope. This sentiment, combined with this frame, is often evoked through narrating speech acts, e.g. when talking about the nation "forming a human shield around our NHS" (Johnson 2020ad: 1) in September or with the December remark: "And all the time we have waiting and hoping for the day when the searchlights of science would pick out our invisible enemy (...) – and now the scientists have done it[sic]" (Johnson 2020at: 1). The objective behind the use of narrating speech acts might therefore be to ensure that his narrative is more memorable and persuasive, thereby convincing the audience of his perspective and the resulting conclusions. Although he tends to describe developments or refer to ancient stories rather than making a direct assertion or claim, these narrating

17 There are three instances of the word 'cavalry' in the dataset, all of them in November. Two of these occur on 23 November, albeit on different occasions. The case described here is from Johnson's oral statement to the parliament (cf. Johnson 2020aq), whereas the second, also part of a narrating speech act, is from the press statement to the public at the same date. Their intention is identical: to reassure that progress is being made, and to caution against becoming overconfident: "we can hear the drumming hooves of the cavalry coming over the brow of the hill but they are not here yet" (Johnson 2020ap: 1).

utterances can be classified as assertive speech acts due to his conviction that he is conveying the truth through the use of these metaphorical expressions.

5.4.2.7 Answer

Lastly, in 19 instances of assertive speech acts, Johnson **answers** hypothetical questions that the public may have. In contrast to the circumstances at PMQs (cf. UK Parliament 2024), where members of parliament are entitled to question the prime minister directly, the monological format of his press statements means he is not responding to a direct question in the dataset. Instead, he is addressing issues that have been raised by the media, the opposition, constituents or in other discussions that are not specifically identified. In this dataset, one instance concerns the case of the policy adviser Dominic Cummings, who broke lockdown guidelines. He addresses the issue by himself raising a pointed question as to whether there is one set of rules for citizens and a second, more flexible one for those in government positions: "Have we been asking you to make sacrifices, to obey social distancing, to stay at home while some people have been basically flouting those rules and endangering lives?" (Johnson 2020q: 1). By proactively addressing a concern likely to be shared by many, this move appears to demonstrate his connection with the general public and attempt a de-escalation of the situation. Despite this initial impression of a proactive approach to the problem, the answering utterance, however, is a lengthy and meandering attempt to justify the adviser's decision:

> "I take this matter so seriously and frankly it is so serious that I can tell you today I have had extensive face to face conversations with Dominic Cummings and I have concluded that in travelling to find the right kind of childcare, at the moment when both he and his wife were about to be incapacitated by coronavirus (...) [a]nd when he had no alternative, I think he followed the instincts of every father and every parent. And I do not mark him down for that. (...) I believe that in every respect he has acted responsibly, and legally, and with integrity, and with the overwhelming aim of stopping the spread of the virus and saving lives." (Johnson 2020q: 1)

Johnson's answer puts forward his own narrative of the events in question, hoping to rebut future criticism from the opposition or the public, with the intent to allay the ongoing "public outrage and media condemnation" (Davies et al. 2021: 4). By depicting a crisis scenario in which children's safety and health are at risk, while simultaneously emphasising Cummings's good intentions, he tries to alter the public's perception of this issue and make them view it in a more favourable light. In his explanation, the prime minister positions himself as an authority figure delivering the final judgement in this ambiguous situation, thereby demonstrating a lack of humility and failing to respect the existence of established rules governing such matters. His inability to acknowledge that the same situation had been resolved numerous times in a different manner by ordinary citizens further exacerbated the public's already considerable anger and contributed to the adviser's resignation later that year (cf. Walker et al. 2020: 2). However, the prime minister's evasive reaction to the scandal, failure to apologise, and his defence of Cummings's actions led to a sharp decrease in public trust in the government during the second half of May 2020 (cf. Davies et al. 2021: 4). By failing to take proactive measures in this case, he demonstrated a lack of concern for the feelings of his constituents (cf. Spyridonidis et al. 2022: 687). This translated into a growing distrust within the public for his capacity to manage the crisis, which is clearly highlighted by Davies et al.'s meticulous tracing of public trust (and distrust) (cf. Davies et al. 2021: 6, see also Seargeant 2023).

In other instances of addressing rumours, the phrase "I know there has been some debate about" (Johnson 2020am: 1) is frequently used as an introductory device, thus reflecting the prime minister's connectedness with the public or, in some cases, the House of Commons, as well as his attempts to counter criticism from the opposition.

A second instance of answering concerns the end of the second lockdown. Here, he can only reply that it will hopefully not be too long before this takes place (cf. Johnson 2020ak: 3). In this statement, Johnson appears to be articulating his genuine feelings, which also resonate with those of the broader public. This indicates his affinity with ordinary British citizens and highlights his recognition of the limitations of his own knowledge. Furthermore, it also demonstrates his reliance on the guidance of scientific experts and the evolving data as he cannot give a clear timeframe for the end of this measure. This concession may prompt the audience to view the prime minister in a favourable light, given his apparent honesty, humility and willingness to seek expert advice. Conversely, it might also evoke perceptions of weakness and uncertainty due to the lack of clarity about the path to resolving the crisis, potentially implying a lack of resolve. Other answers to self-posed questions, 14 of which occur in the autumn period from late September to November, include statements that summarise counterarguments to proposed policies, such as "I know there are many in the House who are concerned about [the policy]" (Johnson

2020am: 1), which is typically followed by reassuring and explanatory speech acts. Johnson's selected proactive engagement with potential inquiries from the public highlights his efforts to project an image of transparency, authenticity and connection to citizens or other elected representatives. Additionally, these speech acts may be interpreted as attempts to neutralise the opposition by depriving them of ammunition on the topics in question, given their previous opposition.

5.4.2.8 Assertive speech acts – summary

Assertive speech acts are typically neutral in tone and convey information in an objective manner. The speech acts 'state' and 'update', which together account for almost 20% of assertive speech acts, mostly provide details about the crisis situation and its progression. They are often accompanied by figures and graphics, which the prime minister references in his statements. In combination with explanations, they embody the informative function of crisis communication and account for a collective total of 52% of the assertive utterances. By giving information regarding the unfolding events and explaining the government's measures, Johnson is ensuring that the public is informed about recent developments and what to anticipate in the future, thereby providing them with a feeling of control and stability. Concurrently, he contextualises the information simple and, in some cases, abridged manner that is comprehensible for citizens, even if they lack a scientific or medical background. By employing a straightforward, clear and confident approach, the prime minister attempts to establish credibility and authority, while also reassuring the public that the situation is being managed by a competent government advised by renowned scientists. These elements appear to be of particular significance in his communication strategy during the securitizing phase of the pandemic, as they constitute over half of his assertive speech acts in the dataset.

The second major subset of assertive speech acts is that of 'affirming' utterances, which, along with 'reporting' speech acts, frequently include announcements of progress. These utterances, which collectively account for nearly 40% of this category, insist that previous policies were successful, sometimes even despite current data that suggests otherwise. This approach often includes calls to continue previous policies, regardless of any current challenges with this approach. The prime minister's explicit commitment to executing the originally designed strategy and the established priorities serves to reinforce his image as a dedicated and reliable leader, even in the face of initial setbacks. This not only demonstrates his strategic capabilities but also provides reassurance to the public, thereby mitigating potential feelings of panic and anxiety. Johnson's arguments are framed in a way that makes his position appear to be the only valid one and suggests that he is conveying an unquestionable truth. Consequently, his language attempts to leave little room for dissent or criticism, and effectively asserts the incontestability of his position. The speech acts in the dataset concerned with giving examples reinforce this impression as each of them contributes to an image of successful government management. They illustrate the leader's capacity to address local concerns while simultaneously managing the pandemic on a national scale. Additionally, they showcase examples of progress and government effectiveness. Building on the prime minister's reassuring tone in the previously mentioned subcategories, the frequency of speech acts giving examples aims to instil a sense of confidence by conveying that the situation is under control. The use of simple and matter-of-fact language in these statements helps to send a message of competence and successful crisis management, thus leading the discourse and asserting authority.

However, the function of 'narrating' speech acts is different. In contrast to the clear and direct utterances found in the other subcategories, these statements are characterised by evocative language and descriptive details, similar to his language as a journalist prior to becoming prime minister. Although a minor speech act, accounting for only 5% of assertives, the use of memorable and vivid imagery allows the speaker to influence the audience in two ways. On the one hand, it improves the audience's capacity to retain the information conveyed due to the distinctive presentation style. On the other, it aids in embedding the prime minister's perspective of current events or scenarios within the audience's cognitive framework by engaging their imagination and emotions, thereby achieving a persuasive effect. The compelling narrative thus makes his messages more impactful and relatable.

5.4.3 Commissive speech acts

Commissives were identified in 206 instances. The smallest utterance has 29 characters, the largest 2,568 characters including spaces, which constitutes the longest individual speech act in the entire corpus. On average, commissive speech acts cover 219 characters (cf. figure A5).

They can be divided into three subcategories: 'promise action', which is divided into six further elements, 'warn' and 'threaten'. Figure 10 provides an overview of speech act distribution within the category of 'commissives'.

Figure 10: Subcategory percentages within the category 'Commissives' in the JPanC20

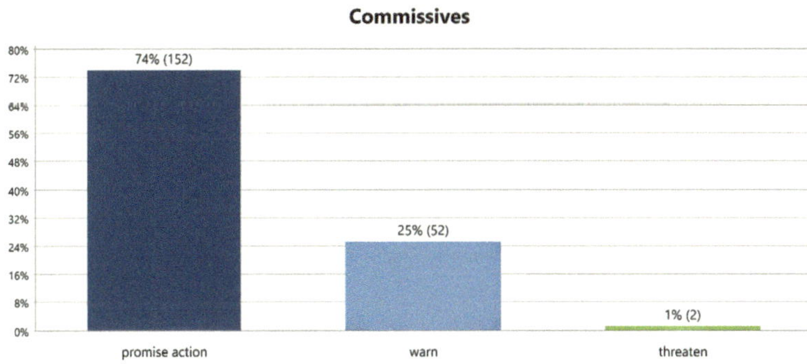

5.4.3.1 Promise action

The most frequently occurring subcategory in commissives is '**promise action**', accounting for 152 speech acts. At 74% of the entire category, this represents a substantial majority. These are utterances in which the prime minister commits his government to action. This subcategory can be subdivided into six parts: 'promise', 'rely on science', 'commit himself', 'imply', 'vow' and 'offer'. Figure 11 illustrates their distribution.

Figure 11: Speech act distribution within the subcategory 'promise action' in the JPanC20

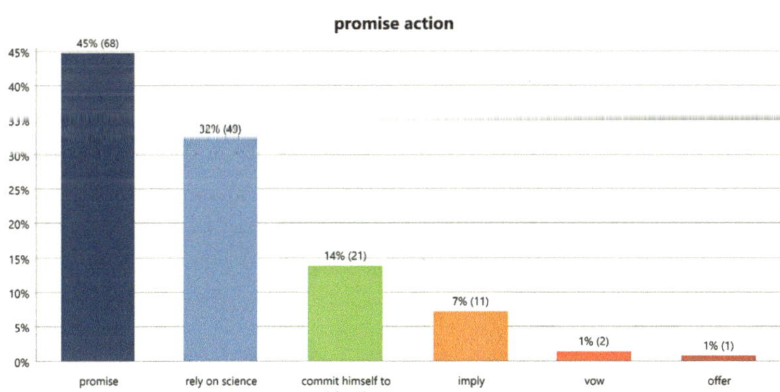

The most prevalent subcategory is '**promise**', of which 68 instances were recorded. Typically initiated with the nodes 'we+will' or 'we+are going to' in combination with a planned action, these utterances are characterised by declarations of intent. In most cases, they refer to increases in the financial resources available for specific demographic groups, e.g. those who have lost their jobs due to the closure of businesses. However, this subcategory is occasionally also used to suggest the future (non-)implementation of particular measures or policies, e.g. a full-scale lockdown. Consequently, the pronoun 'we' usually refers to the government. One example of such a promise of action is the following statement from October 2020: "Nobody affected by this will be left to fend for themselves. And we will expand our unprecedented economic support to assist those affected by these decisions" (Johnson 2020ag: 2). Johnson conveys the image of a government committed to supporting those affected by the closure of businesses, regardless of the financial implications. Despite the absence of a precise definition of the group in question or the particular kind of assistance that will be provided, his clear intention is to reassure the worried audience. Similarly, the use of the modal verb 'will' conveys a strong sense of commitment and assurance. It signals to the public that the government is determined to provide support and that the described actions are not merely possibilities but rather definite plans that the government has committed itself to implementing. Promising "unprecedented economic support", the prime minister once again reiterates the exceptional nature of the ongoing crisis, which has necessitated a significant increase in the level of financial support. The statement offers the reassurance that no individual in need will be left without assistance, in particular emphasising the expansion of substantial economic measures to support those affected. This proactive engagement is designed to instil public confidence and reduce anxiety, while also projecting an image of the government as responsible, assertive and compassionate.

One event that is notable for the high number of promises is the prime minister's Economy Speech of 30 June 2020, which features ten instances of this speech act. On this occasion, Johnson presents his vision for the country and declares his intention to allocate financial resources to a variety of sectors, including infrastructure, zero-emission housing and the health system. He lists an anaphoric series of promises regarding the government's planned post-pandemic actions, which are presented in a systematic, passionate and detailed manner, most of them starting with 'we will':

> "We will continue and step up the biggest ever programme of funding the NHS and we won't wait to fix the problem of social care that every government has flunked for the last 30 years[.] We will end the injustice that some people have to sell their homes to finance the costs of their care (...) [.] We are finalising our plans and we will build a cross-party consensus[.] We will look after those who have looked after us and (...) We will build the foundations now for future prosperity[.] [sic]" (Johnson 2020x: 4f.)

This speech, which resembles an oath rather than a political programme of realistic proposals, presents an ambitious vision for the nation's future. Johnson vows to rectify the shortcomings that have been overlooked by previous legislatures, even extending an implied invitation to the opposition to participate in this endeavour. Once more, he uses the pronoun 'we' to signify the government, making himself appear as part of a dedicated team. His open promises, delivered without hedging, indicate a considerable degree of ambition and a willingness to be held accountable, which illustrate the government's confidence in its capacity for efficacious implementation. At the same time, it signals to the public just how confident the prime minister is in his party and the government.

Similarly, in his address to the General Assembly of the UN, he employs seven promising speech acts. The prime minister pledges financial contributions for the development of vaccines and other health-related technologies, as well as for international scientific collaborations, e.g. in the context of the British G7 presidency in 2021 (cf. Johnson 2020ae: 3). While the content of his promises is similarly ambitious, he begins his sentences with 'we are going to', which signals a less definitive tone than in the previous example and indicates that the proposed initiative is still in the planning phase. In this example, 'we' can refer both to the government and to the United Kingdom as a country. By highlighting the commitments made by the UK, the prime minister aims to demonstrate his country's leading role in the global response to the pandemic. At the same time, it might encourage other leaders to also contribute substantially to the initiative.

The second most frequent speech act within the subcategory 'promise action' is the assurance that the government's actions are **relying on scientific or medical advice**, with 49 mentions. The assertion that all measures are taken in accordance with the most recent scientific data constitutes approximately one third of all speech acts within this subcategory. Johnson regularly asserts that the government is closely monitoring the recommendations provided by experts, which in turn implies that the measures in place represent the best solution: "At all stages, we have been guided by the science, and we will do the right thing at the right time" (Johnson 2020c: 2). To reinforce his argument, he frequently employs graphical representations or numerical data on presentation slides during press conferences to illustrate the numbers discussed, subsequently advocating for the implementation of a corresponding course of action. His commitment to science-based action is illustrated by the frequent presence of scientists at his press conferences. They typically provide input on the current situation, either before, after or intermittently during his speeches. One example is the presence of the Chief Medical Officer, Professor Chris Whitty, at the press conference on 9 September, who is announced as follows: "I will first hand over to Chris to take us through the latest data before I set out how we are responding to it. (...) Thank you Chris. It is clear from that very powerful graphic that we must act" (Johnson 2020ac: 1). This type of introduction, preceding the actual message of the press conference, is typical of the British prime minister during the analysis period. He assumes the role of a host for the accompanying scientist or doctor, allowing the expert to explain the new developments in an evidence-based and technical manner. Following the guest's contribution, Johnson resumes his role as speaker by contextualising and framing the scientific information within the context of broader policy decisions.[18] This strategy not only leverages the experts' credibility to foster trust with the audience but also enables Johnson to reaffirm his leadership position by incorporating expert insights into the government's strategic narrative. Furthermore, it establishes a connection between the government's actions and scientific findings, which are treated as neutral data, and therefore presents him and the ministers as an executive body rather than decision-makers. This might succeed in deflecting responsibility for the conclusions reached and the extensive measures imposed, as they are depicted as absolute necessities rather than as the result of political strategy. It can also help to limit criticism by presenting the decisions as the best possible way of dealing with the situation. The objective of this speech act is, therefore, to provide

18 This "pandemic mantra" (Kirby 2023: 1) of unquestioningly following the advice prompted by scientific data and their projections has been the subject of considerable criticism in the aftermath of the pandemic. Ultimately, it has been labelled a "millstone" (ibid.) on the government's ability to make informed decisions.

reassurance to the public, while simultaneously presenting the government as a responsible and science-based entity that should not be criticised.[19]

The next, comparatively minor element within the subcategory 'promise action' is '**committing himself to doing something**', which accounts for 21 speech acts. They show Boris Johnson making promises that are binding on him as an individual rather than on the government as a collective entity. For example, at the end of September, prior to the implementation of the second lockdown, Johnson asserts: "At this critical moment, when I know people will be wanting to know the details, I will be providing regular updates through these press conferences" (Johnson 2020af: 2). He is committing himself to providing updates on progress and new developments, thereby offering a detailed account of what they will entail. His stated reason, the desire of the public, presents him as being in tune with their needs and striving for transparency. It is, however, noteworthy that he has not specified the frequency of his planned appearances. Furthermore, he employs temporal deixis to indicate that his readiness to increase the regularity of his press conferences is due to the pivotal nature of the situation, implying that this is a temporary state. In contrast to his Scottish counterpart, First Minister Nicola Sturgeon, who provided daily updates throughout the course of the pandemic (cf. Bol 2020: 1), Johnson opts to communicate with the public on a far less frequent basis. Tomkins (2020) condenses the physical absence of the prime minister into the succinct question "Where is Boris Johnson?" (2020: 331), summarising the lack of presence and leadership felt by many Britons in early 2020.

In the subcategory 'promise action', only 14% of speech acts demonstrate a personal commitment to further action (cf. figure 11). Comparing this to the

19 It should be noted that this strategy of hiding behind the UK's traditional "status as a scientific powerhouse" (Imran and Ahmed 2025: 251) received considerable criticism. Paton (2021) delivers a scathing verdict on this approach claiming that both "political leaders and chief advisory scientists blundered big-style" (Paton 2021: 1978) and the government "hid behind the facile slogan, 'following the science', until it was apparent even to its most docile supporters that this was a farcical claim" (ibid.: 1976). Horton (2023) echoes this sentiment, highlighting the government's "inability to understand scientific data (...) and to consistently underestimate the scale and pace of the challenge" (2023: 2277). Spyridonidis et al. (2022) provide a concise summary of this overall impression: "Johnson's hubris, arrogance, anti-science viewpoint, and incompetence at managing and leading (...) drove the emergence of an inappropriate form of leadership (...)[:] an incompetent authoritarian leader in time of a crisis" (Spyridonidis et al. 2022: 691).

77% of promises that refer to the entire government, it can be observed that Johnson rarely makes commitments on a personal level, preferring to speak on behalf of the government as a whole. In absolute numbers, there are around 75 occasions of 'we will' in the initial subcategory of commissive speech acts – 70 of which refer to the government and only five to the British nation – whereas he employs the construction with the first person singular in only seven utterances.[20] The occurrence of these speech acts is relatively infrequent during the summer months, with the final instance taking place on 20 October. Consequently, their cessation occurs during the period of the second lockdown, with a subsequent shift in focus to the government and its measures. The data thus suggests that, in periods of acute political crisis, the prime minister tends to adopt a more cautious approach, avoiding the assumption of personal responsibility for planned actions. This appears to manifest in a preference for maintaining a lower profile and operating within the parameters set by the collective authority of the government, rather than assuming an active and individual leadership position with personal accountability.

There are an additional six instances of speech acts that can be categorised as 'committing himself to doing something' while explicitly placing emphasis on his role as prime minister. In May, he twice alluded to his determination to defeat the virus and begin the community's recovery from the ordeal of the first lockdown. By emphasising his title and invoking a general consensus, he presents himself as a key figure offering a perspective on the way forward. In July, on the other hand, he commits himself to a review of the planned measures, citing his responsibility as prime minister for the security of the nation as the rationale for postponing the complete elimination of restrictions (cf. Johnson 2020aa: 2). Similarly, six weeks later, he declares the 'Rule of 6', proclaiming: "as your Prime Minister, I must do what is necessary to stop the spread of the virus and to save lives" (Johnson 2020ac: 2). In particular, the latter two instances demonstrate that he refers to his role as a defensive measure, arguing that his sense of responsibility for the country necessitates the implementation of longer or stricter measures. He presents himself as being unhappy about the measures he is implementing yet asserts that, in light of his role and accountability as prime minister, he is unable to disregard their necessity.

20 This trend is reflected in the entire dataset with 259 instances of 'we+will' in comparison to 18 cases of 'I+will'.

Lastly, the three November instances of this phenomenon appear to serve another purpose. Acknowledging the difficult demand he had made with the announcement of the second lockdown, Johnson appears to evoke his position to justify this measure, which was perceived as harsh by many in light of the regional diversity in infection rates. To defend his declaration of the second lockdown, he highlights the potential for massive fatalities, stating that, as the person responsible for the welfare of British citizens, he simply cannot accept this loss of life: "But as Prime Minister, when I am confronted with data that projects our NHS could even collapse, (...) I can reach only one conclusion: I am not prepared to take the risk with the lives of the British people" (Johnson 2020am: 1)[21]. Emphasising the responsibility for citizens' health and safety that comes with his role, he presents the severe restrictions as the only viable solution. Additionally, his phrasing allows for a more promising outcome than initially anticipated yet emphasises that Johnson is not prepared to take risks in this regard. Instead, following a cautious approach indicates that he is acting responsibly and with foresight, being aware of the significant responsibility entrusted to him by the citizens he serves. Consequently, the reference to his office can be regarded as a defensive strategy to circumvent criticism and stress the weight of his decisions.

There are three minor speech acts within the subcategory 'promise action': 'imply' with 11 occurrences, 'vow' with two and 'offer' with one instance in the dataset. The instances of **implying** suggest something without stating it outright, as illustrated by the following example: "I am afraid that no responsible PM can ignore the message of those figures" (Johnson 2020ak: 1). Just as in the 'committing himself' example above, Johnson is once again presenting himself as a responsible politician forced to take a hard, but unavoidable decision. He is implying that any criticism of his interpretation of the relevant data is unreasonable and misguided as he is simply acting in a responsible manner, thereby discouraging dissent and reinforcing his own image as a trustworthy authority acting on scientific evidence.

---

21 Statements like this provoked significant consternation within scientific and medical communities assessing the government's crisis management, as the protracted implementation of stringent measures resulted in a substantial increase in infections, and in consequence, fatalities (cf. Binding and McGuinness 2020: 1; Imran and Ahmed 2025: 243; Lilleker and Stoeckle 2021: 6; Pearse 2020; Mason 2020), particularly among minorities (cf. Tomlinson 2026: 160).

The majority of these 11 utterances pertain to either current or forthcoming measures. The admission of an error is implied on only one occasion, in the case of the closure of educational establishments. In light of the government's objective to minimise the impact on education, the prime minister was tasked with striking a balance between the safety of students and the provision of in-person learning opportunities. The statement from 28 May claims that the government is now taking action to rectify the situation, which means reopening schools, and therefore implies that issuing the closure order had in some sense been a mistake: "Closing schools has deprived children of their education, and as so often it is the most disadvantaged pupils who risk being hardest hit. On Monday we will start to put this right" (Johnson 2020s: 3). This marks one of the few instances in the dataset in which one of his own mistakes is acknowledged by Boris Johnson. In this case, the government is the subject of the sentence and is performing the commitment to "put things right", rather than Johnson himself. Nevertheless, the statement appears to be based on flawed logic. Despite acknowledging that the most disadvantaged pupils had been affected most severely by the recent measures, he proposes a phased reopening of educational institutions in which age is the criterion for progression, rather than the level of disadvantage. In any case, the objective of this statement seems to be to demonstrate to the public that he is an honest and responsible individual acting with genuine concern for the well-being of the nation, particularly with regard to the educational access and opportunities available to children.

Vowing was identified as a more pronounced form of commitment, manifesting itself in the form of resolute language. This phenomenon was observed on only two occasions within the *JPanC20*. The press conference from 31 July provides one example: "I cannot – I won't stand by and allow the virus to cause more pain and heartache in this country" (Johnson 2020aa: 2). This utterance displays a strong commitment to addressing the threat and an absolute determination to succeed. The use of the first person pronoun 'I' suggests that Johnson is making a personal commitment and not speaking on behalf of the government in this instance. He presents himself as a determined and active fighter, taking a proactive role in confronting the virus and shielding the nation from harm. However, he does so without delineating the specific means by which this may be attained nor the envisaged outcome itself, thereby affording himself flexibility in determining his approach. Such a heroic statement may reassure the public and inspire confidence, as they perceive the prime minister to be doing his utmost to protect them. This utterance therefore serves to highlight the government's dedication while simultaneously establishing specific expectations for the outcome. Successfully fulfilling this vow has the potential to greatly enhance the prime minister's political capital, thereby reinforcing his image as a strong and effective leader. Conversely, a failure to meet this expectation could result in public disappointment and a significant loss of trust. This makes it a potentially risky speech act in this context. Additionally, this specific speech act may garner particular interest from the media as it represents a relatively unconventional political statement that is likely to draw heightened attention to the issue. This could prove beneficial for the prime minister, as his message will be disseminated more widely and reach a wider audience. However, it may also result in heightened expectations and increased pressure from the media to fulfil the pledge.

Similarly, in the second instance of a vowing speech act in the dataset, in October, Johnson emphasises his determination to stop the spread and effects of the virus, painting himself as a heroic and responsible leader who is particularly concerned with the fate of British children (cf. Johnson 2020ak: 1). Any criticism of the measures imposed is again dismissed as callous and without regard for citizens' hardship, thus invalidating it in advance. This statement therefore once again portrays the prime minister as a dedicated and impassioned politician who is fighting for the common good.

The only occasion on which Johnson **offers** something is at the beginning of the so-called 'second wave' at the end of September 2020. He is committing the government and scientific advisers to respond to questions from the House of Commons with greater frequency and to share more data with members. Furthermore, an invitation is extended to them to participate in daily telephone conferences with the Paymaster General (cf. Johnson 2020ad: 4). With this offer, he is attempting to persuade members of parliament of the necessity for continued vigilance in light of the ongoing threat. Sharing the information on which the government bases its decisions may serve two purposes. Primarily, it enables the dissemination of information regarding developments within the constituencies of members of parliaments, thus facilitating a comprehensive understanding of the situation. This is a fundamental requirement for the implementation of effective political action and therefore a sensible proposition, not only in the context of a pandemic. However, the second objective might be to discredit criticism of the government's measures. At the time of this utterance, there was already a strong probability that the crisis would become more serious with the onset of winter. Johnson may have perceived the need to cultivate a favourable relationship with members of parliament, given his potential need for their support in the event of the introduction of new restrictions. By addressing their queries and providing them with the information they require now, he can reasonably expect to benefit from their goodwill at a later stage. Furthermore, by openly disclosing the offer he has made to members of parliament, he demonstrates his commitment to transparency and willingness to collaborate, thereby portraying himself as a politician dedicated to the public interest.

5.4.3.2 Warn

The second subcategory is the speech act '**warn**', which occurs 52 times. The danger that Boris Johnson most frequently warns about, with 27 explicit statements, is breaking the rules. These warnings are typically situated within a context of reminding the public of the continued threat posed by the virus to their collective well-being, including their way of life and everything that is dear to them. In this regard, the NHS represents a key reference point, with the prime minister warning about the risk of overwhelming the British medical infrastructure on eight occasions. His warnings can be seen as variations of the following statement, released on 4 November: "[Adhere to the rules!] Otherwise we face a bleak and an uncertain future of steadily rising infections and admissions until as I say the capacity of the NHS is breached" (Johnson 2020am: 2). Moreover, he frequently praises the majority of the population for their careful and compliant behaviour before turning to the few who are breaking the rules and issuing a reprimand. In addition to addressing the medical and organisational implications, he also outlines the introduction of increased fines and a greater police presence in public spaces to ensure adherence to social distancing and mask-wearing regulations. His aim is clearly to discourage any deviation from the established regulations by highlighting the potentially catastrophic consequences for the British way of life – including the NHS system and its values – which people are accustomed to and wish to restore.

The second most frequent focus of warnings is the high virality of COVID-19, which is addressed 24 times. Given the unparalleled nature of the pandemic and its rapid progression at the time, he frequently emphasises that the government's response will be contingent upon the evolving situation. In particular, the prime minister highlights the potential implications for the NHS and its patients as a key area of concern: "[I]f we let the lines on those graphs grow in the way they could and in the way they're projected to grow, then the risk is that for the first time in our lives, the NHS will not be there for us and for our families" (Johnson 2020ak: 2). The subject of the sentence, 'we', refers to the British public, thus including the audience and the speaker himself. In the initial section of this utterance, he employs the active form of the verb in combination with a NATURE frame, evoking the image of a plant and portraying British citizens in the role of gardeners, as having the capacity to influence infection rates. It is their responsibility to contain the uncontrolled growth appearing on infection rate graphs, which could have a significant impact on the operational capacity of the NHS. This situation is described as representing a considerable risk as it could result in a scenario where there are insufficient medical resources for the people who are currently listening to the speech. Johnson is thus illustrating the potential implications of rising infection rates on an individual level, emphasising how they could affect everyone, either directly or indirectly through a lack of resources for their loved ones. Given the crucial role of medical care in a pandemic, in addition to the high status of the NHS in British society, this warning appears quite drastic. The phrase "for the first time in our lives" intends to convey the gravity of the situation and the singular circumstances the nation is confronted with. It vividly illustrates the explosive nature of the situation and may also serve as an effective motivator for citizens to adhere to the current regulations, thus supporting the NHS's ability to function and meet its obligations.

This example occurs at the press conference with the most warnings, which took place on 31 October, a mere five days before the beginning of the second lockdown. On this occasion, Johnson issues six warnings regarding the probable and harsh consequences of infection rates at that time, explicitly outlining the serious effects on care staff in hospitals, patients, the elderly and the general population. He asserts that "unless we act we could see deaths in this country running at several thousand a day [-] A peak of mortality alas far bigger than the one we saw in April" (Johnson 2020ak: 1). By using the first lockdown as a basis for comparison, which was widely perceived as the "most stringent restrictions seen in Britain since the end of World War II" (Picheta 2020: 1), he demonstrates the gravity of the situation and the urgent need for decisive action, such as implementing another lockdown. It is presented as the most reasonable measure and the only remaining option with explanatory warning speech acts, as all other measures "still would not be enough, because the virus is doubling faster than we could conceivably add capacity" (Johnson 2020ak: 2). If left to run its course, "doctors and nurses would be forced to choose which patients to treat[,] Who would get oxygen and who wouldn't[,] Who would live and who would die[sic]" (Johnson 2020ak: 2). Painting a grim picture of a situation in which medical personnel are forced to triage patients and issue death verdicts,

Johnson claims that the lockdown is the sole remaining viable option. In an attempt to illustrate the necessity of this stark measure, he reminds his audience that those who may eventually succumb to the illness in this potential future are not limited to the elderly. Simultaneously, the prime minister emphasises the importance of compliance with the strict limitations. Acknowledging the lack of other options to mitigate the predicted development, he identifies the pressing need to prepare the British public for the tough measures and to reinforce their indisputable necessity. The speech act that immediately follows the aforementioned warnings is the declaration of the lockdown: "From Thursday until the start of December, you must stay at home. You may only leave home for specific reasons" (Johnson 2020ak: 2). Given the explicit warnings issued by the prime minister regarding the drastic situation, the act in question can only be seen as a logical consequence of his previous statements. The accumulation of warnings on this occasion therefore demonstrates his intention to persuade the nation of the gravity of the situation, as well as highlighting the necessity of the lockdown in an attempt to encourage compliance with the regulations.

5.4.3.3 Threaten

Lastly, **threatening** speech acts represent the third, very minor category of commissives. In contrast to the warnings described above, threats do not contain the modal verbs 'could' or 'would', which convey a more hypothetical or polite tone. Instead, they rely on 'will' to express a firm and unequivocal certainty about the occurrence of the stated consequence, emphasising its inevitability if certain actions are not taken. This linguistic choice underscores the assertive and often coercive nature of threats, aligning with their function of compelling compliance or action. An examination of the dataset reveals only two instances of threatening speech acts.

The first, concerning businesses, occurs on 25 May. After praising the number of businesses complying with the regulations and thus doing their best to protect employees and their customer base, the prime minister emphasises the government's authority to enforce cooperation if necessary: "While the vast majority of businesses will want to do everything possible to protect their staff and customers, I should add that we will, of course, have the powers we need to enforce compliance where that is required" (Johnson 2020r: 2). The subject in this case refers to the government, illustrating the speaker's role and power as prime minister. With this not very subtle remark, he reminds business owners about the crucial importance of cooperation, irrespective of their personal opinions or sentiments regarding the implemented measures. Employing this threat, he is strongly encouraging them to cooperate voluntarily and offer their support in order to facilitate the achievement of the government's strategic objectives, implying his determination to use all powers available to ensure this.

The second threatening speech act occurs in October, approximately two weeks before the second lockdown, when infection rates in the Greater Manchester area are increasing. Manchester's mayor had not been responsive to the government's suggestions regarding the implementation of a very high alert level, which would have entailed local lockdowns. This anxious situation culminated in the prime minister making the following threat: "Of course if agreement cannot be reached, I will need to intervene in order to protect Manchester's hospitals and to save the lives of Manchester's residents" (Johnson 2020ah: 2). In this instance, Johnson is committing himself to a comprehensive intervention in response to a persistent lack of cooperation from the local administration. Using the first person pronoun 'I', he displays his personal interest in the case and expresses his intention to get involved. The construction "I will need to intervene" implies that he feels forced to do so, out of concern for the city's hospitals and residents. In addition, it highlights his power and position of authority within the government. Johnson once more invokes the necessity of safeguarding the NHS as the rationale for his decision and the implementation of more stringent measures. This indicates a strong sense of duty towards citizens and conjures up the image of a dedicated, impassioned prime minister who wants to keep them safe. As his rather authoritarian statement pertains to the well-being of the city's residents and as such seems to be motivated by a concern for human lives, this position is one with which it is difficult to disagree. The mayor's concerns, however, are not elaborated upon in the context of this utterance nor is there any indication that they have been acknowledged or understood. Instead, Johnson publicly urges him to finally cooperate, which makes the Mancunian appear to be both stubborn and inconsiderate of the danger that his region is facing. The prime minister's threat is preceded by the specific infection rates for the region and a scientific interpretation of them. Additionally, he uses an imploring speech act, pressuring the mayor to reconsider his stance. Subsequent to this threatening speech act, he states that their collective efforts would be much more effective, thereby attempting once again to nudge the mayor into cooperation (cf. Johnson 2020ah: 2). This framing of unity and cooperation softens the threat. However, it is evident that the local administration will have to engage with the government in order to maintain their authority and autonomy. As other regions have been more willing to cooperate once confronted with their high infection rates, the prime minister does not deem it necessary to publicly threaten their local leaders. With the second lockdown looming, he seems to recognise the urgent need to lower infection rates and thus opts to publicly challenge the Mayor of Manchester as the most effective way to intensify the pressure. Simultaneously, this could be intended as a cautionary signal to other local politicians that this is not a time for self-promotion. However, as they are only used twice in the dataset, threats are not characteristic of Johnson's style as a political leader during the crisis.

5.4.3.4 Commissive speech acts – summary

The role of commissive speech acts is of moderate importance in the corpus of UK press statements by Boris Johnson, comprising only 16% of all speech acts. Of these, those classified under 'promise action' constitute the largest proportion, representing approximately three quarters of the total. They represent the prime minister's efforts to reassure the public by pledging government support for several groups significantly impacted by the pandemic. In most instances, he speaks on behalf of the entire government and tends to avoid making personal commitments. However, his various promises regarding the allocation of funds in aid programmes, the introduction of new policies and the relaxation of certain regulations demonstrate Johnson's intention to implement substantial changes to the country. Additionally, they exemplify his confidence in the government's capacity to successfully implement these commitments, conveying a profound sense of dedication and assurance. Except for implying speech acts and utterances that emphasise the scientific basis of decisions, all commissive speech acts can be considered to constitute a proactive commitment on the part of the prime minister. His approach is designed to instil confidence among citizens and alleviate anxiety during the crisis, while also promoting an image of the government as responsible, compassionate and assertive, even when facing criticism.

Johnson appears to place considerable value on the input of his scientific advisers, who frequently accompany him to press conferences. The presentation of statistics and medical data is a common feature of these events and aims to demonstrate that the government's policies are based on scientific observations and recommendations. This information may help to reassure the public and facilitate acceptance of the government's measures and regulations. The advisers' scientific assessments are subsequently presented as an indisputable basis for policy decisions, discouraging potential criticism as unreasonable. On several occasions, Johnson refers to his role as the British prime minister.

By emphasising the necessity of making difficult decisions in light of his responsibility for the entire country, he conveys both passionate concern about the nation and a sense of urgency about the crisis. This context assists in portraying his policies as well-considered and rational decisions, thereby reassuring citizens that Johnson is not taking his responsibilities lightly. In addition, the reference to his position can also be seen as a strategy to discourage criticism, subtly emphasise superiority and portray the opposition as irrelevant, ignorant and egotistical.

It can be argued that commissives can be seen as emotional speech acts as they perform the function of promising to do something, be it with positive or negative intent. The expressions of intention in commissive speech acts usually reflect Johnson's determination to fight the virus and mitigate its effects on the nation. In addition, they demonstrate his genuine concern and sincere care for citizens' well-being, even in instances of threatening or warning speech acts. Together with expressives, they account for approximately half of all utterances in the analysis period, even though they serve a distinctively different purpose in Johnson's crisis communication. It appears that Johnson frequently relies on an emotional-relational communication strategy in this crisis.

5.4.4 Directive speech acts

Figure 12: Subcategory percentages within the category 'Directives' in the JPanC20

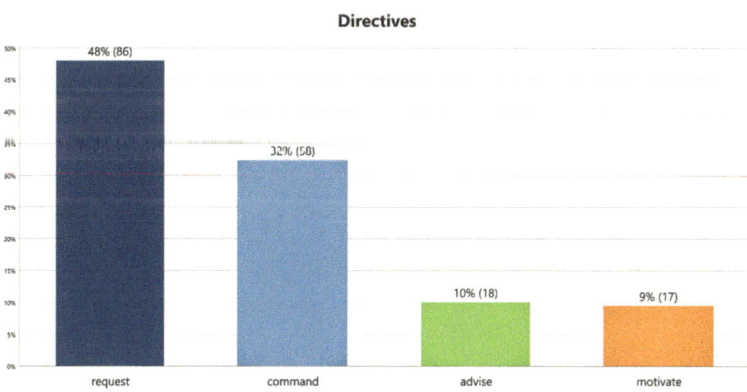

The 179 directive speech acts in the *JPanC20* encompass on average 224 characters including spaces. The largest utterance of this category sees 1,187

characters, where the smallest consists of 20 characters (cf. figure A5). It commands: "And we must act now" (Johnson 2020ag: 1).

Directives can be divided into four subcategories. Almost half of them are associated with the idea of 'requesting' (86 instances), followed by 'command' (58), 'advise the public' (18) and 'motivate' (17). Their distribution is illustrated in figure 12.

5.4.4.1 Request

The most frequent subcategory is '**requesting something**', with 86 instances. In comparison to the second most frequent subcategory, 'command', these utterances appear to be relatively polite as they suggest asking for rather than demanding a desired behaviour. Nevertheless, they are still made with the expectation of compliance and, in this regard, are more forceful than the two minor subcategories of 'advising' and 'motivating' the public. Figure 13 shows the four different speech acts within this subcategory: 'calm/reassure', 'ask you to', 'implore' and 'request'.

Figure 13: Speech act distribution within the subcategory 'request' in the JPanC20

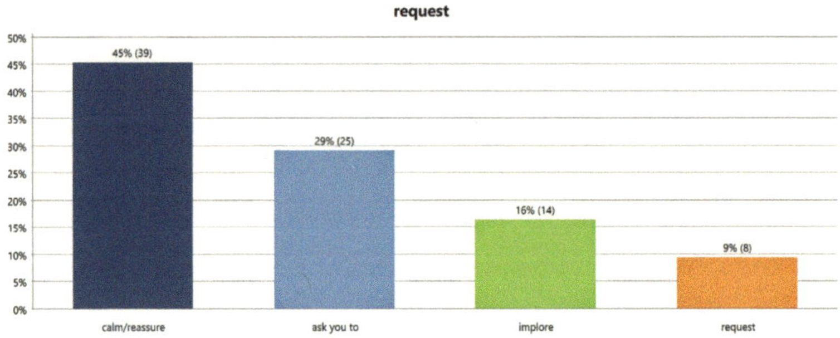

Within the dataset, 39 statements are intended to provide reassurance and comfort to an audience of anxious citizens, urging them not to worry. Those utterances were tagged with '**calm/reassure**', the first element in this subcategory.

In March, Johnson starts out with confident and optimistic comments on the NHS's and the government's preparedness for any potential medical crisis, as well as the low likelihood of the virus impacting the general British population. This quote from 3 March is a typical example of a reassuring statement during the initial phase of the pandemic: "Our country remains extremely well prepared, as it has been since the outbreak began in Wuhan several months ago" (Johnson 2020a: 2). By May, however, his tone shifts to a more cautious approach, with a greater emphasis on the importance of having and following a plan: "We have a route, and we have a plan, and everyone in government has the all-consuming pressure and challenge to save lives, restore livelihoods and gradually restore the freedoms that we need" (Johnson 2020m: 4). The subject in these utterances is the government, which is presented as collectively striving to minimise the impact of the virus on citizens and to facilitate the restoration of their pre-pandemic way of life. In outlining the current priorities, he displays a high level of engagement and authenticity, thereby reassuring the public that the officials' goals align with their own. From September until mid-October, the prime minister reiterates the existence of a roadmap and the progress that has been made since the summer: "We are also, Mr Speaker, better prepared for a second wave, with the ventilators, the PPE, the dexamethasone, the Nightingale Hospitals, and a hundred times as much testing" (Johnson 2020ad: 5). He is attempting to demonstrate to the audience, in this case the House of Commons, that the government is aware of the impending threat posed by the onset of autumn and winter and is taking the necessary preparatory measures. By enumerating the various factors in their favour and even utilising the scientific terminology for some of them, he conveys the impression of being well prepared and knowledgeable about the subject matter. A notable addition during this period is the mention of ongoing community efforts that will positively impact the situation (cf. Johnson 2020af: 2). It places responsibility on each individual member of the public and highlights how they can contribute through their everyday behaviour, rather than solely relying on medical professionals or government action. At the same time, the COMMUNITY frame relieves stress by highlighting that numerous individuals are collectively working towards a positive outcome, each within their respective means. This may provide reassurance to many concerned citizens, while also encouraging them to be active participants in the process.

From November until the last press statement of the dataset on 2 December, the prime minister's focus shifts once more, this time to focus on the recently announced second lockdown. On seven occasions, he tries to reassure the nation that this new lockdown is not as restrictive or open-ended as the first one, which is widely regarded as having had a detrimental impact on the country's economic, social and mental well-being (cf. Johnson 2020am: 2). By stating that the measures are better targeted and more finely calibrated this time, Johnson is emphasising that the country is better prepared for the situation than it was in the spring, while at the same time addressing concerns about the impact on civil liberties and the economy. During this period, his goal seems to be reducing the distress and anxiety that emerged during the initial lockdown. Many citizens experienced significant hardship during this time, including social isolation, financial constraints and mental health issues, which prompted opposition to the second lockdown. By contrasting the two measures in this way, the prime minister's objective is to provide reassurance and give the public a sense of control. This subcategory makes up 45% of requests.

The second element of the subcategory 'request' is termed 'ask you to'. Johnson utilises the explicitly directive speech act of **asking people to do something** on 25 occasions. This relatively polite directive to the public constitutes approximately one third of the subcategory's speech acts. With the exception of four instances, he is asking that citizens comply with a range of rules and guidelines designed to prevent the spread of infection. These directives include maintaining distance, washing hands, avoiding meeting others and being mindful of shielding elderly or vulnerable people. One example is the press statement from 9 September, in which he addresses university students: "Please, for the sake of your education and your parents' and your grandparents' health: wash your hands, cover your face, make space, and don't socially gather in groups of more than 6, now and when term starts" (Johnson 2020ac: 3). He is asking them to comply with current regulations and using the polite 'please', which also adds urgency to his request. The prime minister offers two clear reasons why rule-following is essential. He urges them to refrain from any actions that might jeopardise the continuation of their studies or the functioning of the university, emphasising the collective responsibility of the student body. Additionally, in raising health concerns about their parents or grandparents, he is invoking both familial obligation and empathic concern in an effort to persuade the young adults to act with due responsibility in the coming weeks. By utilising temporal deixis, he underscores the ongoing nature of the threat and the resulting necessity for collective action. The four directives are presented in a concise and clear manner, in the form of a brief and unambiguous list that facilitates both memorisation and compliance.

The other instances of asking for something in the dataset differ slightly. In March, at the beginning of the pandemic, the prime minister requests the return of retired health care professionals to assist in mitigating the pandemic. On three occasions in May, he asks for patience and cooperation from the British public, stating that the government has a reasonable plan in place that would yield results with time. Throughout the first year of the pandemic, however, the essence of Johnson's requests remains overwhelmingly consistent: He encourages the British people to adhere to the current regulations and exercise caution.

The third element of the subcategory 'request', **imploring** speech acts, appears 14 times. The majority of them employ the phrase 'I urge' when addressing the public, with the specific addressee being either a subset of the general public or the entire British population. This can be observed, e.g. in the context of the first lockdown: "And therefore I urge you at this moment of national emergency to stay at home, protect our NHS and save lives" (Johnson 2020i: 3). The use of this verb by Johnson highlights the gravity of the situation and the strength of the appeal, which is further reinforced by the key term 'national emergency'. This phrase, unique within the dataset, may evoke historical connotations associated with World War II and the Blitz or devastating natural disasters, all of which are connected to ideas of grave danger, resilience and determination. The historical and emotional implications of this can inspire a feeling of solidarity and patriotic duty among the audience, prompting individuals to comply with the prime minister's demands as part of their contribution to the national effort. Parts of the slogan 'stay at home, protect the NHS and save lives' are often employed in this context. It was first introduced in March as a simplified directive and subsequently underwent multiple modifications to reflect the evolving pandemic situation (cf. Nartowski et al. 2020: 48; Walker 2021: 1). Here, it serves as a reminder that each citizen can contribute to the collective endeavour in a meaningful way through very simple actions.

Although occurring infrequently in general, imploring speech acts are employed with greater frequency at critical moments during the first year of the pandemic. In March, with the nature of the threat posed by COVID-19 still largely undetermined, the prime minister urges the British public three times to adhere to the published guidelines and to prioritise their own safety and well-being, as well as that of their fellow citizens and the National Health Service. In June and July, the strict rules are gradually relaxed, and his objective seems to be to caution against hasty overconfidence. This period accounts for another third of the imploring speech acts, similar to March, which indicates that this topic is of recurring importance to Johnson. The final four instances are distributed between the end of October (two) and the beginning of November (one) and December (one). Here, he attempts to reassure the audience and to encourage them not to panic, instead urging them to engage in constructive cooperation by following the established regulations and measures.

The last element of this subcategory, the speech act '**request**' itself, accounts for eight instances. These comprise the prime minister's requests for collaboration and support. Approximately half of these statements are directed at the general British public, in which he asks for active support of the government's efforts (cf. Johnson 2020aa: 1), with another addressing the council leaders of the Greater Manchester region in a plea to finally collaborate. The last three are directed towards other statesmen and stateswomen at the United Nations General Assembly, who are asked to facilitate cooperation and free markets by lifting export controls and tariffs on vital goods for fighting the pandemic. This shows that cooperation is not only desired on a small scale within regional communities but is also demanded in a global sense. However, this appears to be a minor speech act within the 'requesting' subcategory of directive speech acts.

5.4.4.2 Command

The second subcategory of directive speech acts, constituting 58 speech acts, is **commands.** It is further subdivided into three parts. The first, 'command', accounts for approximately three quarters of this subcategory, with 'instruct' making up the remaining quarter. Furthermore, one single instance of 'prohibit' can be identified. Their precise distribution is visualised in figure 14.

Figure 14: Speech act distribution within the subcategory 'command' in the JPanC20

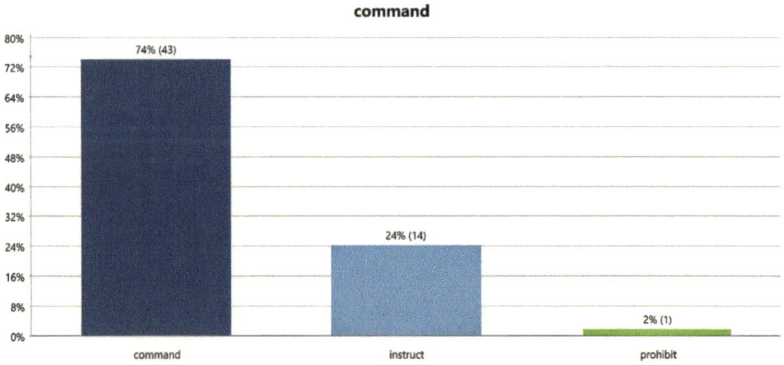

The first element, '**command**', can be identified in 43 instances. These speech acts are characterised by the nodes 'you/we+must' or 'you/we+need to', respectively.[22] In the majority of cases, the addressee of Johnson's calls for action can only be determined by considering the context. The conduct expected from citizens mostly involves adherence to the new rules, such as: "[i]f you test positive with one of these fast new tests, then you must stay at home" (Johnson 2020ah: 3). As evidenced by this example, the language used is straightforward, comprising basic vocabulary. The desired actions are presented in a comprehensive manner, summarising numerous individual situations with a brief instructive sequence of simple and logical steps. This sets clear and understandable expectations for behaviour, helping to encourage cooperation and compliance with the established rules. An additional element often associated with the call for proper behaviour is evident in the explanation accompanying the declaration of the first lockdown in March: "From this evening I must give the British people a very simple instruction – you must stay at home" (Johnson 2020i: 1). Despite calling it a "simple instruction", the imperative 'you+must' effectively transforms his utterance into a command. Even though it is an unprecedented order unfamiliar to the vast majority of Britons, the instruction itself is relatively simple and easy to understand. However, in order to emphasise the seriousness of the situation, the prime minister follows up with a threat of police sanctions a few sentences later. This is a common occurrence in this subcategory, as six of his commands are accompanied by a reference to police enforcement. Therefore, this speech act can be considered to be among the more authoritative ones, in which the speaker exercises their authority to instruct citizens on how they should behave.

By contrast, the actions demanded of the government, typically initiated by 'we+must', seem rather complex and lack specificity. One example is Johnson's demand for vigilance in July: "We must be willing to react to the first signs of trouble" (Johnson 2020aa: 1). The indications of said trouble and the subsequent response demanded are not defined in the surrounding speech acts, which encompass a warning, an expression of caution and a statement of the newest figures. As a result, this call for alertness is rather vague, albeit situated in a context of caution and concern. It could serve as a reminder to the public and

22 The sole case of 'you+must+not' is classified under the third part of this subcategory, 'prohibit'.

members of parliament to comply with the current regulations and avoid becoming too complacent as the crisis continues to unfold.

Another example of a command directed at the government is the prime minister's speech on the economy and pandemic recovery in June, in which he states: "we must use this moment – now – this interval to plan our response and to fix of course the problems that were most brutally illuminated in that covid lightning flash" (Johnson 2020x: 2f.). Calling on the nation and especially the other members of the executive to seize the moment of respite during the summer, he advocates for collaboration in planning the recovery of the British economy. In addition, Johnson shifts the focus to other pressing issues in British society and politics that have been exacerbated by the pandemic. He uses the metaphor of a 'lightning flash' to powerfully illustrate the idea that the pandemic has illuminated systemic issues, which must now be addressed without delay. The combination of this moment of opportunity and the sudden realisation of deficiencies makes his command appear even more imperative. Furthermore, the sequential structure of the utterance is maintained in the subsequent speech acts, which present a comprehensive list of areas in which new policies are to be implemented. However, this speech act is preceded by expressions of understanding regarding citizens' concerns about the potential long-term economic impact of the pandemic on the economy and their own employment. Following Johnson's directive, he expresses impatience regarding the sluggish response to certain issues and laments the fact that exemplary British capabilities and institutions are not sufficient to deliver services in a consistent quality and timely manner. The prime minister's statement culminates in a pledge to create a more robust and equitable socio-economic landscape by addressing the long-standing neglect of certain areas and regions. His commanding speech act therefore serves to initiate a collective appeal, directed towards the executive as well as the entire nation, for collaboration in this endeavour. This deliberate and visionary approach to crisis management is a bold attempt to instil confidence in the government's ability to control the virus and plan for the country's recovery. It indicates the government's intention of prioritising other political concerns once the immediate challenges posed by the pandemic have been dealt with and thus introduces the first explicit notion of desecuritization, the third phase of securitization (cf. section 2.2). In addressing the executive branch in this manner, Johnson once again underscores the importance of collaboration and prompt action. In contrast, commands directed at the public seem to reinforce the necessity for compliance with the current regulations.

Instructive speech acts, the second element of the subcategory 'command', occur 14 times. They are used to clarify the conduct expected of the public in the period following the respective press conference and encompass elements such as appropriate behaviour before or during the lockdown, procedures for suspected infections, measures for shielding and interactions with the NHS (cf. Johnson 2020i: 2). These utterances frequently contain the modal verbs 'need to' or 'should' in combinations such as 'you+need to', 'we+need you to' or 'you+should' (cf. Johnson 2020m: 3). Especially during the first lockdown, when the entire situation was novel and concerning, and basic regulations had yet to be established, Johnson employed instructions with great frequency. Consequently, the majority of instructive speech acts are found during the first wave in March, with individual occurrences in May, June, July, October and November. One press statement involving an exceptional sequence of instructive speech acts containing modal verbs was made at the beginning of the first lockdown:

> "That's all – these are the only reasons you should leave your home. You should not be meeting friends. If your friends ask you to meet, you should say No. You should not be meeting family members who do not live in your home. You should not be going shopping except for essentials like food and medicine – and you should do this as little as you can. And use food delivery services where you can." (Johnson 2020i: 2)

In this statement, the prime minister sets out the instructions that the public should follow in order to comply with the lockdown. He presents a list of potential scenarios that citizens might encounter, such as the desire to meet friends or family, and offers advice on the appropriate response. To address the audience directly, the second-person singular pronoun 'you' is used in each sentence. The use of this technique makes the instructions appear more personal than those conveyed in a more rigid and absolute manner, such as "Don't meet friends". In addition, the friendlier tone may encourage compliance with the new rules. The language used is characterised by simplicity and brevity, offering a set of rules that can be readily understood and followed by all. Acknowledging that these behaviours might not be feasible for all individuals at all times, Johnson allows for necessary adaptations by using the phrase "where you can" and employing the more permissive 'should' instead of 'must'. Nevertheless, his message of minimising external contacts remains clear, providing the public with easy guidelines. This illustrates the distinction between commands and instructions. While both are authoritative and intended to be adhered to by the audience, instructions allow for the possibility of disagreement or alternative actions, whereas commands are more assertive and do not permit such flexibility. Instructive speech acts are therefore typically used as a means of providing guidance to individuals in order to facilitate their adjustment to this novel way of life and instil a sense of confidence regarding the acceptability of specific behaviours. The use of straightforward vocabulary and brief, succinct sentences helps to achieve this purpose for all citizens.

The final element of the subcategory 'command' involves prohibiting something. Only one instance of a **prohibition** can be found in the dataset. On 9 September 2020, Johnson states: "You must not meet socially in groups of more than 6 – and if you do, you will be breaking the law" (Johnson 2020ac: 2). This strongly worded prohibition is employed to clarify the recently introduced 'Rule of 6' and to eliminate any potential for misunderstanding or exploitation of loopholes. In the context of a rising number of cases and the growing likelihood of a second lockdown, the prime minister is seeking to mitigate the infection rate through the implementation of this new measure. To emphasise the gravity of the situation, he resorts to the use of the only explicit prohibition in the dataset. Within the scope of this speech, the police and potential sanctions are mentioned four times. Furthermore, he refrains from any form of hedging or ambiguity in this context, in stark contrast to the announcement of other new measures or rules. Consequently, Johnson appears to be profoundly serious and determined in his intention to convey the immense gravity of the situation to the audience.

5.4.4.3 Advise

The third most frequent subcategory, '**advise**', occurs 18 times in the dataset. It comprises utterances that carry less force than the previous two subcategories. In such instances, the prime minister offers guidance to the general public by communicating in a less formal register. One example can be found in his article in the *Mail on Sunday*, published on 7 May: "work from home if you can but travel to work if you can't. And avoid public transport if you can, but use it if you can't" (Johnson 2020p: 2). Rather than prohibiting certain behaviours outright by threatening sanctions, he advises the public while allowing them to determine approaches most effective for them. In this way, he emphasises their accountability while not denying their autonomy. He may be making this concession due to the upcoming relaxation of the strict lockdown measures as this loosening of restrictions came into effect shortly after the article was published. Johnson's advice strikes a balance between caution and an acknowledgement of the necessity of business operations. The modal verb 'should' is frequently used in this context, e.g. "I am afraid that those who have been asked to shield themselves should continue to do so" (Johnson 2020s: 3). This statement, made a few weeks after the example above, acknowledges the increased autonomy and self-responsibility of individuals as measures are relaxed step by step. It implies that it would be prudent to follow the advice given, but if the affected groups decide otherwise, the government respects their decision.

Advising speech acts are predominantly found in March, at the beginning of the first lockdown, when the required behaviour was still novel, challenging and difficult to remember. Many of Johnson's recommendations concern hand hygiene and social distancing, areas where citizens needed help adapting. Nevertheless, in these utterances, he ultimately leaves it to citizens to determine their level of compliance. The number of instances of advice provided in March is nine out of a total of 19, whereas in May, at the conclusion of the lockdown period, four instances are recorded. The remaining six occurrences are documented in September, at the beginning of the second lockdown period. Johnson therefore uses advice in situations where there are significant and critical shifts in expectations, such as lockdowns, with the aim of facilitating compliance on the part of citizens. This subcategory accounts for 10% of directive speech acts.

5.4.4.4 Motivate

The fourth subcategory of directives is called 'motivate' and occurs 17 times. By **motivating** the audience, the prime minister attempts to encourage them to engage in behaviours that he deems essential for combating the spread of the virus. It constitutes the smallest subcategory of directive speech acts, with 17 occurrences comprising utterances that exhibit a relatively low degree of authority. Twelve of these utterances are directed at the British public, whereas two target local leaders and three took place during his speech to the UN General Assembly. The former are all found at the conclusion of the respective press statements and are characterised by their optimistic and engaging choice of words. One example is from 27 April, where Johnson concludes his speech with the following words:

> "I say to you finally if you can keep going in the way that you have kept going so far[,] if you can help protect our NHS to save lives[,] and if we as a country can show the same spirit of optimism and energy shown by Captain Tom

> Moore[,] who turns 100 this week[,] if we can show the same spirit of unity and determination as we have all shown in the past six weeks[,] then I have absolutely no doubt that we will beat it together[,] we will come through this all the faster[,] and the United Kingdom will emerge stronger than ever before[.]" (Johnson 2020l: 4)

Citing the success of previous weeks, which he attributes to meticulous preparation, unwavering resolve and the prevailing spirit of unity among the British people, he expresses his confidence in overcoming the difficult situation. This combination of praise and promise is employed to encourage the audience to maintain their efforts in containing the pandemic. His choice of words is powerfully evocative and is designed to inspire. The reference to Captain Thomas Moore, who served as a symbolic figure in the first year of the pandemic, intensifies this effect. Hailed as a "beacon of light through the fog of coronavirus" (Stewart 2020: 1) in the prime minister's proposal to grant him a knighthood, the 100-year-old veteran's fundraising campaign for the NHS embodies the virtues of dedication, perseverance and optimism, which the prime minister hopes to instil in the entire nation.[23] Consequently, Moore is presented as an inspiring role model to encourage the audience. The concept of collective identity as a motivational tool is also evident in two other speeches where he urges citizens to unite and to remember that they are not alone (cf. Johnson 2020i: 3; Johnson 2020ak: 3).

The remaining three cases of motivating speech acts at the UN General Assembly follow the same strategy, albeit with a different intention. His primary objective appears to be the fostering of collaboration and the reduction of barriers between nations. This is exemplified by his advocacy for the elimination of tariffs on essential medicinal products (cf. Johnson 2020ae: 4). Furthermore, he promotes investment in the COVAX initiative, a project aimed at developing vaccines and distributing them to countries lacking their own (cf. World Health Organization 2023). Moreover, Johnson proposes the establishment of a global network of research centres to identify and contain potentially dangerous pathogens before they reach pandemic levels. His objective is to foster enhanced cooperation and dialogue between nations. The prime minister attempts to encourage the other assembly members by outlining the advantages and disadvantages of non-cooperation: "Unless we unite and turn our

23 He was knighted in July 2020 by Queen Elizabeth II and is thus referred to as Captain Sir Thomas Moore afterwards.

fire against our common foe, we know that everyone will lose. The inevitable outcome would be to prolong this calamity and increase the risk of another. Now is the time (...) for humanity to reach across borders and repair these ugly rifts" (Johnson 2020ae: 1). In contrast to the motivating speech acts directed at the British audience, the choice of words is less straightforward here, and the overall tone is less optimistic and framed in a more negative way. It seems that fear is leveraged as a motivating factor to encourage international collaboration, capitalising on the present opportunity and first insights gained from this pandemic. In his speech, three instances of motivational speech acts are identified, occurring at the beginning, in the middle and towards the end. This example is the first and may not fulfil its full motivational potential, as Johnson employs it as a prompt to initiate discourse on other subjects, including the international vaccine initiative. He concludes his address with a series of optimistic motivational sentiments, such as: "Though the world is still in the throes of this pandemic, all these steps are possible if we have the will. They are the right way forward for the world" (Johnson 2020ae: 4). The tone of this utterance is consistent with those discussed above, emphasising that strength comes from unity and collaboration, which reflects the speaker's intention to encourage countries to work together. Motivating speech acts constitute only 9% of all directive speech acts, making them a relatively minor subset of this category.

5.4.4.5 Directive speech acts – summary

Directive speech acts are of moderate importance in the *JPanC20*, making up only 14% of all speech acts, a proportion similar to commissives. This indicates that the prime minister tends to avoid the use of an authoritarian communication style in favour of a more indirect approach in the dataset[24]. Directives seem to serve a dual purpose: They instruct British citizens to adhere to the new rules while simultaneously encouraging their participation in the collective efforts to fight the virus. Within this category, the most prevalent types of individual speech acts are reassurances – a subset of requests – and commands, each occurring around 40 times. Johnson thus prioritises the task of reassuring the nation and providing clear instructions on how they should act.

---

24 This conclusion is drawn solely based on speech acts coded in the dataset. Nevertheless, other scholars have identified Johnson's leadership style indeed "characterised by authoritarianism, heroism, populism, and fragmentation" (Spyridonidis et al. 2022: 690, see also Paton 2021: 1974; Binding and McGuinness 2020: 1).

Setting forth clear behavioural expectations for citizens in combination with speech acts mitigating feelings of anxiety and panic may increase the likelihood of substantial collaboration and assistance. His orders indicate that the government is aware of the urgency of the situation and the threat to the nation. Concurrently, however, Johnson's straightforward directives and his advice grounded in scientific principles convey the impression that the government is responding in a prompt and appropriate manner. Providing the public with advice represents a relatively minor aspect of directive speech acts, accounting for merely 20 instances. It allows Britons to determine their own course of action based on the scientific guidance provided by the government, tailored to their individual circumstances or requirements, thus trusting their willingness to contribute to the collective effort. Motivating speech acts are found on 17 occasions, providing encouragement to the public and fostering their sense of collective strength and resilience. Johnson employs a combination of praise for progress achieved and the promise of success to encourage the audience to maintain their efforts in containing the pandemic. This is achieved through the use of positive role models, such as Captain Sir Thomas Moore, who are intended to inspire the audience and reinforce the importance of continued effort in the face of the ongoing pandemic. The prime minister's requests, commands and advising speech acts aim to foster collaboration in combating the virus's spread and mitigating the pandemic's effects on the country.

When addressing the public, Johnson employs the strategic use of concise and accessible language, ensuring that his messages are comprehensible to the widest possible audience. This linguistic simplicity increases the likelihood of compliance with his directives. A notable distinction emerges when these speech acts are contrasted with utterances directed to an audience of fellow politicians, such as those delivered at the UN General Assembly. In such instances, the choice of words appears to be considerably more sophisticated, incorporating elaborate metaphors, rather complex vocabulary and historic or religious references. This approach, unconstrained by the need to be universally comprehensible to the British public, is probably intended to convey a sense of cosmopolitanism and to enhance the memorability of the message.

5.4.5 Declarative speech acts

Declaratives are the smallest category in the dataset. The largest individual speech act from this category encompasses 2,567 characters including spaces, whereas the smallest only has 32 characters: "But it is now a global pandemic"

(Johnson 2020c: 1). On average, utterances from this category consist of 493 characters, the largest value in this corpus (cf. figure A5).

Only 98 occurrences can be attributed to this speech act, which account for 8% of the total dataset. This category is made up of three subcategories. 'Announce measures', the largest, comprises 63 utterances, followed by 'declare something' with 26 instances and 'lift measures' with nine instances. Figure 15 provides an overview of the three subcategories.

Figure 15: Subcategory percentages within the category 'Declaratives' in the JPanC20

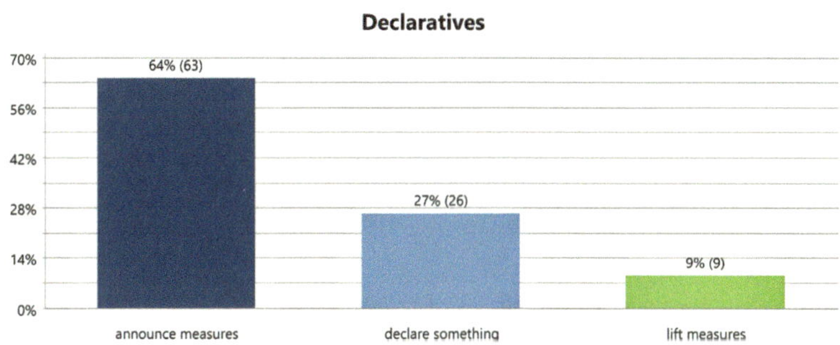

5.4.5.1 Announce measures

Figure 16: Speech act distribution within the subcategory 'announce measures' in the JPanC20

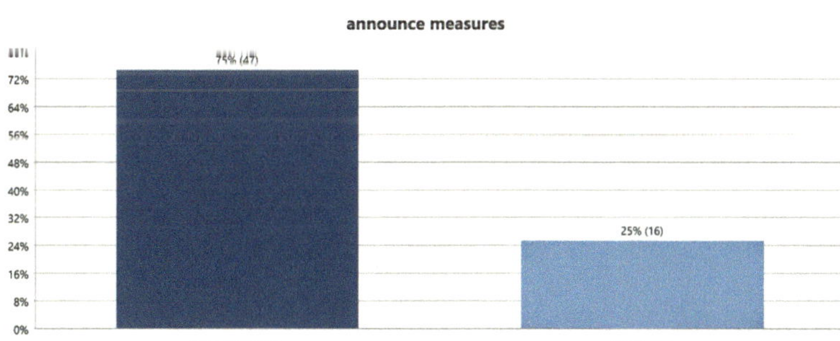

The majority of declarative speech acts, 63 utterances in total, take the form of '**announcing new measures**'. This subcategory is divided into the two elements 'issuing a new policy' with 47 instances and 'imposing rules' with 16, as illustrated in figure 16.

The first element comprises 47 instances of the prime minister **issuing a new policy**. These encompass broader strategies for achieving the overarching goals set out by Johnson, such as the implementation of support bubbles (cf. Johnson 2020v: 3), local restrictions (cf. Johnson 2020ag: 2) or the beginning of a new lockdown (cf. Johnson 2020ak: 2). However, this kind of speech act is not only used for communicating stricter or increasingly robust measures but is also employed for replacing measures, effectively lifting them. Following the introduction of five new policies in March, a total of 16 speech acts are recorded in May referring to a variety of policies. These include the establishment of a system of five alert levels, new guidelines for retail and steps for reopening schools. Five instances are again documented in June and July, respectively, indicating progress towards the easing of restrictions. No instances of this particular speech act were found in August, which may be due to a combination of the low incidence rate and the low number of press releases during the summer holiday period. In September, five new declarations are issued concerning travel quarantines, contact tracing and the restriction of opening hours, indicating a new surge of cases. This culminates in the announcement of the second lockdown on 31 October, preceded by three speech acts in the first part of October. November sees six occurrences, three of which appear in one press statement on 23 November, introducing the new tier system. The two December press statements in this dataset also each contain one instance of this element, again referencing the tier system. The month of May thus represents a notable exception to the established pattern of policy announcements, which typically occur at a rate of approximately five per month.[25] This significant outlier, with more than triple the usual number of declarations, probably reflects the need for stable guidelines during the gradual relaxation of lockdown regulations amid uncertainty and cautious optimism. It seems likely that Boris Johnson recognised the need for more declarations in order to provide citizens with structure and reliable guidelines, thereby encouraging them to exercise restraint and avoid excessive enthusiasm. The language used in these declarations is generally assertive and in 31 of the 47 utterances in this subcategory,

25 December has been excluded from this observation as its two days are not representative of a whole month's frequency or pattern.

the modal verb 'will' is employed to describe the new reality with these policies in place. The use of this construction in place of hedging or modal verbs that convey a degree of tentativeness, such as 'should' or 'might', expresses certainty and assertiveness.

The two press statements where this speech act is most frequent, with four occurrences each, are issued on 9 September, when he introduces the 'Rule of 6' (cf. Johnson 2020ac: 2f.), and 10 May. In this latter statement, the new system for categorising alert levels in the context of the ongoing pandemic is introduced. The new strategy is announced by outlining the underlying structure of the policy:

> "the lower the level the fewer the measures. The higher the level, the tougher and stricter we will have to be. There will be five alert levels. Level One means the disease is no longer present in the UK and Level Five is the most critical – the kind of situation we could have had if the NHS had been overwhelmed. (...) thanks to your sacrifice we are now in a position to begin to move in steps to Level Three." (Johnson 2020m: 2)

Once more, the syntax is characterised by the use of concise sentences without subordinate clauses. The use of comparative adjectives in the parallel structure 'the lower...the fewer, the higher... the tougher and stricter' facilitates the understanding of the concept. This conditional structure emphasises the logical consistency underlying the five levels of the new policy and the severity of the measures. Basing decisions on objective criteria further reinforces the image of the prime minister as a rational and deliberate leader. His vocabulary in this utterance is relatively simple and avoids the use of complex linguistic structures in an attempt to facilitate comprehension among the British public. The implementation of a numeric alert system demonstrates a transparent approach, enabling the audience to easily understand the varying degrees of risk and the corresponding measures. Using 'will' in describing the new policy makes it appear real and once again discourages criticism. Overall, the linguistic choices are designed to enhance understanding, to emphasise the gravity of the situation and prepare the public for potential escalations in response measures.

This statement also exemplifies the distinction between 'issuing a new policy' and the second speech act in the 'announce measures' subcategory, termed 'imposing rules'. While the former is associated with the introduction of general strategies, as illustrated by the given quote, the speech act **imposing rules** concerns the implementation of specific and more detailed rules at the individual level. The following statement further illustrates this distinction: "Border Force will step up enforcement efforts at the border to ensure arrivals are complying with the quarantine rules" (Johnson 2020ac: 3). Here, Johnson announces that police at the border will ensure that new arrivals are in compliance with British quarantine rules – an utterance that would fall under 'issuing a new policy'. He does not provide a detailed account of the specific regulations that must be adhered to. Consequently, he is outlining a policy, but not the precise and detailed procedures for individuals travelling, which would fall under the second speech act, 'imposing new rules'.

In a total of 16 utterances, he imposes new regulations. About half of these are implemented in March, coinciding with the initial lockdown. At this time, the prime minister appears to feel compelled to clarify expectations for citizens to ensure more widespread compliance. Given the extent of the implemented changes, which entail a significant departure from the nation's established routines and conventions, it is essential to provide clear and unambiguous guidance on the desired new behaviour. To achieve this, the prime minister presents a series of scenarios in which non-essential contact should be avoided. Among the key recommendations he outlines are the following:

> "people will only be allowed to leave their home for the following very limited purposes: shopping for basic necessities, as infrequently as possible[;] one form of exercise a day – for example a run, walk, or cycle – alone or with members of your household; any medical need, to provide care or to help a vulnerable person; and travelling to and from work, but only where this is absolutely necessary and cannot be done from home." (Johnson 2020i: 2)

Johnson's statement is designed to clearly communicate the strict constraints on future movements and activities. His syntax is straightforward and repetitive, closely resembling an itemised list with bullet points. Similarly, the vocabulary of this speech act is relatively simple and avoids any technical terms. The lexical choices, including 'only', 'very limited', 'as infrequently as possible' and 'absolutely necessary', reinforce the strictness of the announced measures, presenting them as non-negotiable. To illustrate the narrow range of acceptable reasons for being outside, he offers several examples of acceptable forms of exercise with the intention of reducing ambiguity and discouraging a nonchalant approach to these limitations. By mentioning the permitted "one exercise per day", he illustrates the practical consequences of this new regulation for citizens' daily lives, helping the extent of the demands to sink in. The passive voice in the phrase "will only be allowed" conveys a sense of requiring authorisation, thereby suggesting associations with authority and control. The statement is thus presented with the objective of explicitly articulating the strict limitations on public movement and activities going forward. The use of authoritative language in combination with a structured syntax and restrictive vocabulary enables the prime minister to communicate the gravity of the newly implemented policy in a clear and unequivocal manner. Using illustrative examples and precise qualifiers helps to clarify the narrow boundaries of permissible actions, thus ensuring that the audience fully understands the impact of these restrictions. The declarative nature of the utterance reflects the authority behind them, indicating that this announcement is binding and non-negotiable. These two speech acts, 'issuing a new policy' and 'imposing rules', both fall under the subcategory 'announcing new measures', which accounts for 64% and therefore constitutes more than half of all declarative speech acts.

5.4.5.2 Declare something

The two remaining speech acts within declaratives are relatively minor. On 26 occasions, Johnson is explicitly '**declaring something**'. This illocution performs the change of status of something by uttering the corresponding words, which is rather uncommon in the dataset. It constitutes a form of governmental authority that is particularly reflective of executive power. Prior to the beginning of the first lockdown in March, two cases can be identified in which Johnson declares new rules of behaviour that Britons are required to follow. He emphasises the necessity of safeguarding the NHS from being overburdened, maintaining the continuity of educational institutions and protecting the elderly from the virus as it is particularly dangerous for them (cf. Johnson 2020c: 1f.). In line with the specified premises, the government proceeds to enact its policies over the following weeks. In May, three declarations are issued concerning the prospective course of action, namely the reduction of regulations for citizens, accompanied by a gradual lifting of the restrictions. This approach also enables the government to define the form and conditions of progress, which are beneficial when it comes to presenting itself in a favourable light. The declarations in September are part of a speech delivered to the United Nations General Assembly in which the British government outlined its priorities, including providing financial support to the COVAX initiative and fostering international cooperation. One important instance in the dataset occurs on 31 October, when the second lockdown is announced: "there is no alternative. From Thursday until the start of December, you must stay at home. You may only leave home for specific reasons" (Johnson 2020ak: 2). This utterance represents one of the few instances in this corpus where a declaration is combined with another speech act, as it simultaneously imposes new rules. With this statement, a new phase of the pandemic is initiated. The prime minister's statements effectively cancel all plans Britons had for the coming weeks, whether for leisure, business or long-standing commitments. Instead, they are forced into a state of enforced isolation within their own homes. This significantly reduces citizens' autonomy in exercising their free will and agency. Consequently, this speech act constitutes a highly significant act with far-reaching consequences for economic and social structures, as well as for Britons' daily lives. Johnson's declaration therefore marks an abrupt transition into a new stage of the pandemic in which the public is placed in a state of enforced compliance, deviating from the previous state of relative normality with minor limitations.

While the given example may encompass directive utterances, its principal function is that of a declarative, as it brings about a transformation in the status of the situation. Moreover, while the measure in question may have been approved by the House of Commons, it is through this press statement that citizens are first made aware of these far-reaching restrictions. Consequently, the announcement effectively enacts the measures at the moment of its utterance, thereby constituting a declarative speech act.

Although the term 'lockdown' itself is avoided, the measures announced by the prime minister are largely similar to those implemented during the first lockdown in March. His clear and unambiguous language demonstrates the gravity of the situation and leaves no room for misinterpretation. 'Lockdown' is employed in the final paragraph in a manner that is both dismissive and contradictory: "We are not going back to the full-scale lockdown of March and April, it is less prohibitive and less restrictive, but from Thursday the basic message is the same: Stay at home. Protect the NHS. And save lives" (Johnson 2020ak: 4). It can therefore be concluded that Johnson's strategy is to implement a lockdown without explicitly using that unpopular term.[26] The contrastive structure of this utterance provides reassurance to the audience that, while the new restrictions are serious, they are not as severe as before, which might mitigate potential resistance or anxiety. Employing the imperative form in combination with the phrase "there is no alternative" implies inevitability and finality in an authoritative manner, with the distinct implication that any opposition or dissent is discouraged. The use of the modal verb in "you may only leave home for specific reasons" allows for limited exceptions to this strict new rule. However, the restrictive language, indicated by 'only', highlights that exceptions to this rule should be considered as unusual and are only permissible in narrowly predefined cases. The temporal deixis situates the restrictions in time, thereby providing clarity regarding the timeframe in which the rules are applicable. Together, these commands simplify a complex situation into a straightforward, actionable directive that the audience can readily recall and implement.

Furthermore, eight declarations can be identified in November, followed by four in the two December statements. While the November instances concern the tier system and supplementary funding for relief programmes, the statement released on 2 December marks the announcement of the first approved vaccine for the United Kingdom:

> "today we can announce that the government has accepted the recommendation (...) to approve the Pfizer-BioNTech vaccine for distribution across the United Kingdom. after months of clinical trials, involving thousands of people to ensure that the vaccine meets the strictest, internationally recognised, standards of safety, quality and effectiveness.[sic]" (Johnson 2020at: 1)

The government had positioned the vaccines as an essential milestone in the long months in which "humanity has been tormented by COVID" (Johnson 2020at: 1), signifying the beginning of the final phase of the pandemic. Consequently, the approval of this vaccine marks a pivotal moment in the journey

26 A similar phenomenon was observed during the announcement of the first lockdown, even though the employed speech acts were distinctively different. He avoided any declaration with the term 'lockdown' and rather gave a direct order, "you must stay home" (Johnson 2020i: 1), which was followed by explanations about the causes and consequences of this unprecedented measure for the public. An indication of the dread Johnson feels with regard to lockdowns gives the utterance from 22 October, in which he calls it a 'Scylla' after the mythological monster.

towards controlling the virus, offering a pathway towards a return to normality and demonstrating the government's effectiveness in this endeavour. Johnson highlights the exceptional quality of the vaccine, which adheres to the highest international standards for safety and efficacy. This further aims to instil confidence among the public with regards to the vaccine's safety, despite its accelerated production. In a surprising display of objectivity, his announcement immediately acknowledges the contributions of all parties involved in this success. The use of formal language, evident in verbs such as 'announce', 'accepted' or 'approved', conveys the information in an official manner. The stark contrast between this formally worded statement and his usual expressive tone highlights the authoritative nature of the declaration, drawing attention to its content. The effect is further intensified by the utterance at the beginning of the press statement, which establishes the tone with a metaphorical representation of prolonged anticipation: "all the time we have [been] waiting and hoping for the day when the searchlights of science would pick out our invisible enemy [and](…) give us the power to stop that enemy from making us ill – and now the scientists have done it" (Johnson 2020at: 1). This metaphor evokes vivid images of defensive strategies employed during nighttime operations in the Second World War. It draws a parallel between the current pandemic and a war situation in which the country is under attack and needs to act in a defensive manner. Scientists are portrayed as relentless in their pursuit of the enemy and as ultimately responsible for saving the nation by empowering its defence. The description of the scientific research behind the vaccines as "a kind of biological jiu-jitsu" (Johnson 2020at: 1) contributes to this WAR frame with creative fighting techniques and images of struggle, illustrating Johnson's appreciation for the pioneering and challenging nature of the work. Concurrently, it indicates the considerable pressure that he and the entire nation are experiencing due to the prevailing economic, social and mental challenges. This declaration therefore acts as a fundamental turning point during the pandemic, completely changing the government's strategy. Instead of focusing on immediate crisis management, the government is now pursuing a strategic and deliberate approach to guiding the country into a post-pandemic era. This impression is reinforced by the concluding speech act in the press statement, which expresses relief: "we are no longer resting on the mere hope that we can return to normal next year in the spring, but rather on the sure and certain knowledge that we will succeed: and together reclaim our lives and all the things about our lives that we love" (Johnson 2020at: 3). This statement, which can be described as almost triumphant, conveys the clear sentiment that this challenging phase is now finally coming to a successful conclusion. Although he employs the first person plural as a member of the British public rather than as a representative of the government or in his capacity as prime minister, Johnson's palpable relief in this utterance reflects the significant pressure and stress associated with his role and responsibilities. By claiming the success for the nation, he seeks to foster a sense of unity and solidarity by indicating that all Britons contributed to this collective achievement – not just scientists, government officials and medical professionals but also ordinary citizens who adhered to the prescribed measures. Moreover, the conjunction 'we+will' displays resolve and confidence in his actions, thereby offering the public a sense of assurance and security. The use of the pronoun 'we' and the emotional tone contribute to a sense of cooperation and optimism, as opposed to the authoritarian tone employed in the earlier formal declaration. This contrast underscores the official status of the announcement. The objective of this communication strategy may have been to provide reassurance to the public by making the shift in policy stance clear. This development occurred at a critical moment when public morale was low as a result of months of lockdowns, restrictions and uncertainty. By announcing the availability of a vaccine in this way, the prime minster intends to restore hope and reassure the public that the end is in sight.

Consequently, declarations are infrequent in Johnson's crisis communication, occurring mainly when new phases in the pandemic's development are initiated. These phases may be characterised as either positive, such as the start of the vaccination campaign, or negative, such as an increase of restrictions. Additionally, a commonality of all declarations is that the prime minister presents these utterances as absolute truths, without the use of conditionals or hedging, thereby discouraging criticism or dissent by framing the declaration in an absolute manner. Instead, there are multiple instances of combining 'we+will' or 'will+be', which showcases determination and authority. The final declaration pertains to vaccine acceptance and represents one of the most eagerly anticipated milestones, which was conceptualised as the beginning of the pandemic's final phase. The use of formal language in the declaration at this juncture highlights its significance.

5.4.5.3 Lift measures

'**Lifting measures**' is the smallest subcategory of declaratives, with only nine instances. Closely related to the aforementioned speech act of declaring something, the presence of this minor speech act is contingent upon the prior implementation of a rule. It can be found in seven press statements that were published during two distinct periods: The first spans May to July 2020 and the second comprises the final week of November and the first days of December. Its lexis is comparable to that of the previous subcategory, although the content differs. A considerable number of instances of the modal verb 'can' appear in the introductory sentences preceding the announcement of rule relaxation. The following example illustrates this phenomenon: "we can't do anything for swimming pools but we can do something for lakes and the sea. and this is where we can go significantly further because there is a lower risk from outdoors than indoors[sic]" (Johnson 2020n: 3). The prime minister's alternation between 'can' and its negation 'can't' presents the government as being constrained by external factors, suggesting that delaying rule relaxation is not a matter of willingness but is contingent on other factors. This is probably a reference to scientific advice, particularly in light of the comments concerning the "lower risk". The contrastive structure of the phrase emphasises the positive news of allowing free exercise under certain conditions. The statement continues with the actual rule-lifting speech act:

> "So from Wednesday there will be no limits on the frequency of outdoor exercise people can take. You can now walk, sit and rest in parks, you can play sports and exercise, and you can do all these things with members of your own household, or with one other person from another household, provided you observe social distancing and remain 2 metres apart from them." (Johnson 2020n: 3)

He is providing citizens with a clear indication of the date on which the measures will come into force and the exact activities that are now permitted, thereby giving citizens a sense of security. The high frequency of 'can' indicates a shift in the status quo. Focusing on what is possible rather than on what is still prohibited allows for a more constructive framing of the situation, motivating the public with the visible progress that is being made. Subsequently, the newly permitted activities are outlined in detail, providing citizens with concrete examples that offer reassurance and a sense of security.

The rule-lifting speech act itself primarily features constructions with the node 'we+will', such as in this example from July, when the first lockdown officially ended:

> "from 1 August, we will reopen most remaining leisure settings, namely bowling, skating rinks and casinos, and we will enable all close contact services such as beauticians to resume. (...) We will also allow wedding receptions for up to 30 people. All of these measures for 1 August should be done in a Covid Secure way. In September, schools, nurseries and colleges will be open for all children and young people on a full-time basis, as planned." (Johnson 2020z: 4)

As in the example above, he begins his rule-lifting speech act with a clear timeframe for when the new rules will apply. Phrases, such as "from Wednesday" and "from 1 August" leave no ambiguity and manage public expectations in a transparent way. Simultaneously, they present the speaker as a powerful authority figure with a structured approach to the subject matter. This parallel structure is observed in seven of the nine instances of this specific speech act (78%), which suggests a characteristic pattern. In this example, lifting the rules can be seen as being the exact opposite of the speech act 'imposing new rules', as it also refers to the implementation of specific and very detailed rules at a personal level. Johnson presents an overview of the upcoming changes using a list-like parallel structure. He references various societal sectors and repeats the verbal phrase 'we will+verb+object'. The selected verbs, such as "reopen" or "enable", have an active and positive connotation, thereby indicating the government's capacity for agency and progress. The most common combination within this speech act is 'we will+allow', which occurs five times in the first cluster of this speech act. They appear not only in July but also on 10 June, when the prime minister announced the relaxation of the most severe lockdown limitations (cf. Johnson 2020v: 3). This phrase, and in particular the verb "allow", reiterates Johnson's position within the government and thus highlights his own authority. The use of the active form of the verb in the future tense emphasises the prime minister's proactive and constructive role in facilitating the reopening of society. By using 'will' instead of 'going to', Johnson demonstrates his confidence in the efficacy of these new policies as well as his determination to see them through. Despite remaining cautious, as evidenced by his admonition that the public should conduct themselves safely, the tone of this statement appears upbeat and relieved. His intention may be to both instruct citizens on how they can safely exercise their newly won freedom while also encouraging continued compliance with the regulations by demonstrating their effectiveness.

The three utterances in November and December, however, do not contain the phrase 'we will allow'. Instead, they employ passive constructions, such as "people will be able to leave their home" in the statement from 23 November or "you will no longer be instructed to stay at home" on 26 November, which direct attention away from the government as the body issuing regulations. This shift of focus onto the new reality reduces the perception of governmental authority and depersonalises earlier contentious directives. Johnson's linguistic choice serves to diminish the perception of authoritarianism associated with the preceding policies, instead portraying them as impartial decisions demanded by statistical evidence rather than top-down commands. Additionally, the future modal verb 'will' emphasises the certainty of forthcoming positive changes, while maintaining focus on the respective policy's impact rather than on who was originally responsible for it. These statements lift specific rules, in line with the tiered Winter Plan, but do not constitute a complete reversal of lockdown measures. Therefore, the subsequent speech act can be understood as an expression of caution regarding the ongoing danger or an expression of sympathy for the continued necessity of the measures in place. This decision is once more justified by the necessity of safeguarding the NHS.

The summer instances of this speech act are firmly located in the latter part of the press statement, whereas the three autumn cases are situated in the first half, with one occurring at the beginning and two in the middle. The distinction between the two, also evident in the lexical choices surrounding the subject of the utterances, may indicate a shift in Johnson's strategic approach. While he conveyed the rule relaxations in an optimistic tone during the summer period and emphasised his role in this positive development, his tone during the second period is rather concerned and cautious, reiterating the ongoing threat. This may be associated with the season and the anticipated progression of infection, but it may also reflect the prime minister's increasing familiarity with the pandemic, which prompts him to avoid any premature celebration.

'Lifting rules' constitutes a minor subcategory that is largely concerned with measures implemented during the initial phase of the lockdown. This represents the ultimate objective of Johnson's crisis communication strategy, namely the elimination of all restrictive measures. Given the focus of the dataset on the securitizing act rather than on the subsequent phase of desecuritization, the low frequency of this speech act is unsurprising. Nevertheless, it plays an important role in Johnson's crisis communication strategy, not only as the ultimate goal but also by demonstrating initial successes and providing tangible evidence of progress for the public.

5.4.5.4 Declarative speech acts - summary

Declarative speech acts amount to only 8% of all speech acts. The utterances in this category, the smallest in the *JPanC20*, all feature a similar syntax and lexis. The sentences are predominantly brief and free of multiple subordinate clauses or complex context, which facilitates comprehension of the new policies for the audience. In many cases, an anaphoric structure is employed, which reinforces the underlying logical consistency of the statement. The choice of vocabulary in these speech acts is characteristically straightforward and avoids the use of technical terms or elaborate metaphors. Just as in the case of directives, this linguistic simplicity in combination with the structured approach increases the likelihood of comprehension among the maximum number of audience members and, in turn, the probability of widespread compliance with the measures. Almost all speech acts in this category are followed by expressions of caution or warnings about the ongoing danger.

Most of the declarative utterances announce new measures (64%). The most frequent individual speech act in this category is when the prime minister announces a new policy, which is unsurprising given the events that occurred during the dataset's timeframe. Given the considerable initial infection rates and the rapid surge in cases, coupled with a higher than anticipated lethality, Johnson employs this speech act regularly, averaging approximately five instances per month. May 2020 is the major outlier with 16 instances. During this month, he significantly increases the number of declarations to communicate relaxations in the strict initial lockdown restrictions. These are gradually replaced by more lenient guidelines, contingent on a number of key metrics concerning infections and hospitalisations. The declarations empower the government to define the form and conditions of progress in this phase, which is beneficial for presenting a more favourable narrative. Johnson frequently employs the passive voice in these announcements, thereby conveying associations of authority and granting permission. Simultaneously, he implies that his actions are not driven by personal volition but are instead the result of a process where numerical data and scientific counsel serve as a neutral basis for decision-making.

The second subcategory, 'declaring something', which is of relatively minor relevance in the dataset, changes the status of something. In these statements, which primarily occur when initiating new phases of the pandemic response, Johnson typically distils a complex situation with numerous variables into a simple and actionable directive that the public can easily understand and follow. Framing the declarations as absolute truths, he portrays his decisions as the only possible solution, thereby discouraging criticism or dissent.

The subcategory 'lifting measures', the smallest within this category, is typically initiated by a specific time indication. It constitutes the ultimate goal of securitization: to reduce measures because the threat is being contained. As the period of this dataset is from the beginning of the crisis, a low number of such declarations is expected. Nevertheless, these utterances are essential for the prime minister's crisis communication as they demonstrate the success of the government's policies by providing tangible evidence of progress. This might increase trust and, in turn, enhance public willingness to comply with the restrictions.

This most authoritative speech act displaying the executive power of the government has a minor role in this dataset, thus indicating that Johnson has refrained from adopting an authoritative communication style. However, declaratives have the purpose of providing clarity on the situation by offering unambiguous information about current events and developments. Furthermore, the act of labelling the current phase of the pandemic provides the public with the correct terminology and contextualisation to facilitate informed discussion about the situation, thus reducing the likelihood of misinformation and panic, and serving as a tool to reassure the public. At the same time, these declarations convey a sense of security and control, as the government establishes expectations regarding future actions or the projected timeline. Furthermore, declaratives contribute to the establishment of authority and, consequently, the assertion of control over the situation, which serves to reassure the public that the crisis is being managed effectively and efficiently. During the summer, the use of the active form of the verb in the future tense emphasises the proactive and constructive role of the prime minister in facilitating the reopening of society. In contrast, the autumn period of rule-lifting speech acts focuses on favourable outcomes, such as regaining lost freedoms and the ability to leave home, while the use of the passive voice minimises the government's perceived role in the decision-making process.

5.4.6 Speech act distribution and co-occurrences

Comparing the press statements over time, noticeable differences can be found in the occurrence and frequencies of the individual speech acts. The **press statements with the fewest speech acts** are from 9 March 2020 (cf. Johnson 2020b) and 11 May 2020 (cf. Johnson 2020o), with seven individual speech acts respectively. The former consists of 529 words, representing the fifth smallest in the entire *JPanC20*, while the latter contains 811 words. In comparison to the average of 1,223 words per press statement, the latter statement is comparatively brief, although not among the ten shortest. Consequently, a lower number of words does not necessarily correspond to a lower number of speech acts. Instead, the observed paucity of speech acts may be attributed to the timing. In March, the speaker's perception of a minor crisis necessitating minimal intervention is reflected by the small number of speech acts employed. However, by May, a notable shift towards a heightened awareness of the crisis had occurred. Nonetheless, a swift resolution and post-crisis recovery were still being anticipated and the countermeasures in place were considered suitable, which may have resulted in this small number of speech acts. In contrast, the **press statement with the most speech acts** is Boris Johnson's Economy Speech, with 64 individual speech acts (cf. Johnson 2020x). It constitutes the longest press statement in the dataset with 3,706 words. In this speech, the prime minister provides an evaluation of the government's management of the pandemic to date, details current processes and outlines his plans for the economic future of the country. The high number of speech acts on this occasion is therefore not surprising. Furthermore, the dataset includes a total of 1,271 speech acts across 46 press statements, which averages to a rate of 27.6 per press statement. The distribution of speech acts over the 56,349 tokens yields a **Speech Act-Token-Ratio (SATR)** of 2.25%. This indicates that, on average, each speech act in this dataset consists of 44 words.

The allocation of speech acts across the five categories exhibits an unequal distribution. Expressives constitute one third of all speech acts, with assertives accounting for approximately another 30%. This highlights the prime minister's emphasis on conveying emotions or attitudes, as well as making statements or assertions. Commissives and directives each make up around 15% of all speech acts, while declaratives, at 8%, form the smallest category.

This **finding contrasts with previous studies** on securitizing speech acts during the pandemic. For instance, **Marsen and Ali-Chand's (2022)** analysis of 18 speeches by three South Pacific prime ministers from the first four months of the pandemic found a dominance of directives with about 30% of speech acts, followed by declaratives, which also amount to percentages between 21% to 30%. Assertives are recorded slightly below, with commissives around 15% and expressives being the smallest speech act with 15% in the case of New Zealand, 13% for Australia and only 4% for Fiji (cf. Marsen and Ali-Chand 2022: 9). These numbers may differ because of the timing and size of this dataset, however, as the corpus consists of only six selected speeches per speaker. Additionally, the authors recorded directives, declaratives and assertives as categories but differentiated between two individual speech acts for expressives and three individual speech acts for commissives. This method may have resulted in a distorted image.

Similarly, **Majeed's (2022)** examination of one speech by the president of the United States from March differs from the results in the *JPanC20*. She found predominantly assertives (50%) with declaratives being the second most frequent speech act with 27%. Directives and commissives are both recorded at 10%, with expressive speech acts merely occurring in 0,7% of all annotated utterances (cf. Majeed 2022: 100f.). This study focuses on a single speech, depicting a snapshot of Trump's early communication in the pandemic. It is therefore impossible to determine whether this speech act distribution is characteristic for the entire securitizing move or just due to the selection of this specific speech. Majeed's findings are thus only somewhat comparable.

The most comparable study, conducted by **Schueler and Marx (2023)**, analyses speech acts in the Dutch government's COVID-19 communication from March 2020 to April 2021. Their findings indicate that assertives were the most frequent speech act, comprising more than half of all instances (57%), a pattern also observed by Majeed (2022). Directives ranked second at 15%, followed by commissives at 11%. Expressives account for a mere 7% of the annotated speech acts, while declaratives represent the smallest category at just 3%. With the exception of the role of expressive speech acts, the overall distribution resembles the findings in the *JPanC20*. In particular, the limited significance of declaratives, along with the relatively minor role of commissive and directive utterances, is a shared characteristic of both studies. Moreover, Schueler and Marx's observation that modest directives are more frequently employed than strong directives align with the results of the British case study. The primary divergence lies in the markedly reduced presence of expressives in favour of assertives, which suggest that Johnson's highly expressive and emotive rhetoric may be a unique feature of his securitizing discourse. They do not report on individual speech acts but discuss the distribution of speech act categories over the length of their corpus elements, just as section 6.2 does for the *JPanC20*. However, the corpus for this research is comprised of over 170 speakers, including more than 150 journalists and several members of the Dutch government. This results in a diverse body of speakers, rendering this study only somewhat comparable.

Other studies examining securitizing moves by influential figures, such as in a speech by the UN Secretary-General in an Emergency Special Session on Ukraine, similarly observed a significant number of assertives and directives (cf. AlAfnan and Oshchepkova 2022: 96). In this dataset, assertives amount to 38%, with 'reporting', 'informing' and 'announcing' the most frequent individual speech acts. Directives are found in 36% of all coded utterances. The rather moderate speech act 'requests' is the most frequent individual speech act. Commissives occur only half of this, with the two individual speech acts 'guarantee' and 'promise' each showing four times. The only reported expressives are 'thanking' (two instances) and one act of 'welcoming', which amounts to 6% for this category. No declaratives are observed in this speech.

Consequently, the findings of preceding studies demonstrate a rather diverse distribution of speech act categories. However, the equally heterogeneous selection of analysis periods and speakers hampers meaningful comparisons. The relatively low number of declaratives and directives employed by the British prime minister in the *JPanC20* is therefore unexpected. This distribution may stem from the longer analysis period as well as from the idiosyncrasies of Johnson's colourful and expressive rhetorical style. However, it might also indicate a deliberate effort to refrain from adopting an authoritarian tone in favour of a more relational and emotional approach by Boris Johnson.

5.4.6.1 Frequency distribution of speech acts

In total, 49 different types of individual speech acts can be identified in the *JPanC20*. Explanations constitute the most frequent individual speech act, with a total of 119 occurrences. The second most prevalent speech act, 'acknowledge others', occurs 25% less frequently, with 88 instances. The next most common speech act is the commissive 'promise', occurring at roughly half the frequency of explanations. Figure 17 shows the 20 most frequent individual speech acts, along with their respective categories and frequencies. The illustrated data represent 40% of the 49 different types of individual speech acts found in the dataset, accounting for approximately three quarters (74%) of all coded utterances in the corpus. A comprehensive table of all individual speech acts is provided in the appendix (cf. figure A2).

Figure 17: Distribution of the 20 most frequent speech acts in the JPanC20; sorted by absolute frequency; categories coded by colour: red: expressives, green: assertives, orange: commissives, yellow: directives, blue: declaratives

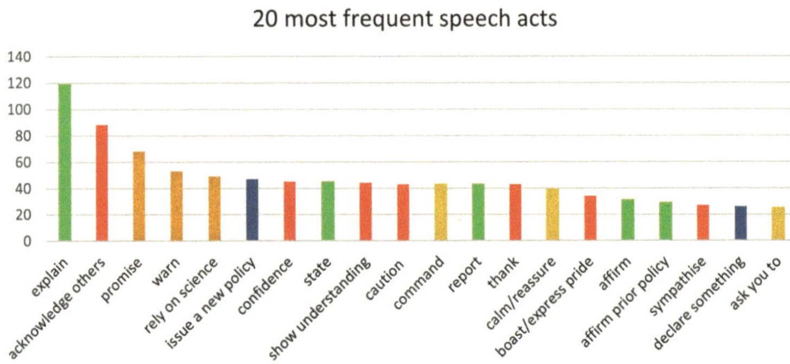

Notably, the **distribution of the 20 most frequently employed speech acts** closely mirrors that of the overall speech act categories in this corpus (cf. figure 2). Expressives, highlighted in red in figure 17, include 324 different utterances and account for 34% of this speech act subgroup. Similarly, they make up 33% of the total number of speech acts. Assertives, indicated in green, account for 267 utterances or 28% of this speech act subgroup. This percentage is comparable to the 29% of all speech acts that they represent in the entire *JPanC20*. Thirdly, commissives, shown in orange, comprise 170 utterances or 18% in this subgroup. This aligns with their overall average of 16% in the corpus. The category highlighted in yellow, directives, is at 11%, or 14% in the entire *JPanC20*. This represents 107 individual utterances distributed across the 20 most frequently employed speech acts. Lastly, declaratives are again the smallest category, comprising 73 utterances in this subgroup, which accounts for 8% of both the speech act subgroup and the entire corpus. The findings on the 20 most frequent speech acts therefore align with Johnson's overarching communication strategy during this phase of securitization, with only a slight reduction in the case of directives. Additionally, figure 17 clearly illustrates the prime minister's emphasis on expressives and assertives, which are featured with seven and five speech acts respectively. Commissives and directives each appear three times in this subgroup. With the former occurring at the upper end of this frequency list and the latter being positioned in the second half, their relevance to the communication in question is already evident. The fact that there are only two instances of declarative speech acts in this subgroup of the 20 most frequent speech acts indicates their relatively minor occurrence in the *JPanC20*.

The speech act utilised most frequently, **explain**, is the only one occurring over 90 times. Its frequency in the corpus indicates a pivotal role in Johnson's securitizing move. It appears that explanations are the primary function of his press statements and can serve three crucial purposes in his communication during the securitizing move. Firstly, to elaborate on the nature of the threat and its extent, and secondly, to explain specific regulations and the corresponding behaviour expected from citizens. Lastly, the third function of this speech act may be to make his reasons for policy decisions more transparent. His emphasis on transparency and the articulation of his perspective is intended to ensure that the public is fully informed of the latest developments and the rationale behind the government's decisions and actions. By adopting an explanatory and, at times, even educational approach, he fulfils the informative function of crisis communication in a way that enables the public to make informed decisions and act in accordance with the specific requirements of the situation (cf. Olsson and Eriksson 2020: 420). By offering explicit and detailed instructions about the desired actions, the behaviours expected of Britons are conveyed clearly and unambiguously, increasing the likelihood of compliance. Furthermore, defining desired behaviours provides reassurance and reduces anxiety during this challenging and uncertain period. This aspect fulfils the instructive and adjustive functions of crisis communication, establishing a direct relationship between the prime minister and the public (cf. ibid.: 420). By cultivating this personal connection, he may also have intended to foster trust and present an approachable image, thereby reducing criticism of his government and instances of non-compliance. Additionally, he is able to direct the public's attention, establishing a certain tone and asserting authority while subtly guiding the national discourse.

The prominence of **acknowledgements of others** as the second most frequent speech act reinforces the idea that this crisis can only be resolved through a collective approach. By explicitly highlighting the contributions of others – including medical or scientific advisers and members of the community – the prime minister both recognises their efforts and implies that responsibility for assisting the government rests with all members of society. This positions Johnson and the government in a leadership role while simultaneously incorporating the general public as an integral component of the collective, requiring their active and decisive involvement in implementing measures to address the crisis, in line with their respective capabilities. Furthermore, this strategy may lend the presented policies and measures greater legitimacy by explicitly referencing the scientists involved. Consequently, the crisis management approach employed by Johnson appears to be both rational and devoid of any ulterior motives.

Promise, the third most frequent speech act, introduces a new element to Johnson's overall communication strategy. Besides explaining the danger, the measures and his decision-making process, and emphasising other actors' contributions, this speech act stresses his commitment to delivering solutions. He presents himself as a suitable candidate for solving the crisis by providing assurances on various issues that have emerged. It demonstrates his willingness to assume responsibility and proactively pursue solutions, and he thus reassures the audience of the government's capacity for action. Additionally, the relatively high number of promises may be characteristic of the securitizing move itself, as it suggests that measures or solutions are not yet fully implemented but are being committed to for future action. This description aligns with the initial phase of securitization. Despite being a relatively small category, this speech act's recurrent presence indicates that the prime minister is a dedicated politician who is so confident in his abilities that he is able to make commitments in place of merely proposing vague plans or stating general intentions. However, the relatively high frequency of promises could also pose certain risks, particularly if they cannot be fulfilled.

In contrast to promises, which tend to focus on positive outcomes initiated by the government, the next most frequent speech act, **warn**, anticipates negative developments. Besides committing the government to action in predefined unfavourable scenarios, this speech act also implies Johnson's emotions. It reflects his emotional state of feeling pressured and alarmed by recent developments, which he shares with the public. Bridging the categories of commissives and expressives, it conveys governmental transparency and authority while simultaneously humanising the speaker through an affective connection with the audience. The nuanced use of this speech act demonstrates how emotional and performative aspects shape Johnson's securitizing act and aim to influence public perception in a manner that fosters compliance.

These four speech acts occur most frequently. The remaining 45 are less common, albeit still relevant for Johnson's communication. They occur less than half as often as explanations and, with the exception of warnings (with 53 instances), are observed fewer than 50 times.

Subsequently, the **correlations between explanations and other speech acts** will be examined. On nine occasions, explanatory utterances correlate with expressive speech acts, with three instances each of expressing understanding and gratitude. Two of the former occur in May and one in September 2020 (cf. Johnson 2020s: 4). Johnson emphasises his comprehension of the challenges inherent in the situation and provides the audience with transparent information regarding the latest developments and their implications, with the objective of making the situation more manageable for them. The three instances of expressing gratitude for the work of others in explanatory utterances occur predominantly in March and May, and take place in the context of working together to mitigate the negative impact of the virus on the community (cf. Johnson 2020ac: 3).

Two of the seven instances of explanations occurring alongside commissive speech acts are documented in May, with the remainder occurring in autumn, specifically three cases on 31 October and two in November. These are primarily warnings (cf. Johnson 2020ak: 2), which the prime minister presents as a direct result of the development in question, as well as assertions that governmental decisions are based on scientific advice. This is one example from the October speech: "Because as you can see from some of those charts, the R has been kept lower than it would otherwise have been, and there are signs that your work has been paying off" (Johnson 2020ak: 1). His statement demonstrates that his executive actions are informed by a scientific approach, grounded in numerical data and its scientific interpretation. This combination may serve to circumvent potential criticism by presenting his actions as objective and informed decisions.

Similarly, seven instances of co-occurrence with directives have been identified, the majority of which involve reassuring utterances. Comments such as "We are not going back to the full-scale lockdown of March and April, (...) these measures are less prohibitive" (Johnson 2020al: 4) assist the public in comprehending the new rules and categorise them as nothing to fear.

Only four statements appear to be correlations of explanations and declarations. All of these utterances are speech acts that impose rules and typically encompass longer passages of information which are then interrupted by brief explanations. The speech from 22 September provides an example, showing the larger speech act of imposing stricter rules being broken up by smaller utterances that explain a detail or the necessity of the restrictions (cf. Johnson 2020ad: 3). This strategy serves to ensure that the audience understands the reason behind the decision for a particular rule, which in turn increases the probability of compliance.

By frequently providing explanations and combining them with other speech act categories throughout the dataset, Johnson attempts to foster transparency and clarity in his communication, with the aim of offering the public a clear rationale for decisions during a period of uncertainty. This approach facilitates the establishment of trust by demonstrating that the government's decisions result from careful deliberation and scientific advice, while simultaneously seeking to mitigate potential criticism. It also helps alleviate public anxiety by rendering complex policies more comprehensible.

5.4.6.2 Frequency distribution of subcategories

Searle's five categories (assertives, expressives, commissives, directives and declaratives) are subdivided into subcategories, which in turn contain individual speech acts (see table A1). In this study, a total of 29 subcategories have been identified. Figure 18 shows the 20 most frequent among them. Once again, the colour of the columns indicates which of the five categories they belong to. Only three subcategories occur more than 100 times in the *JPanC20*, while 11 subcategories see 50 or more coded utterances. These include the columns between the two commissive subcategories in figure 18, 'promise action' and 'warn', which are indicated in orange. The final five subcategories on the right of the diagram each occur a maximum of 20 times.

The commissive 'promise action' constitutes the most prevalent subcategory, with a total of 152 occurrences. The second most frequent subcategory, 'gratitude', appears on 131 occasions and underscores the prime minister's emphasis on collaboration and the notion that the crisis can only be resolved by collective action. The subsequent subcategory is the assertive 'explain'. In contrast to the first two subcategories, this cannot be divided into further subsets but remains an individual speech act. Occurring 119 times, it is also the most frequent individual speech act (cf. section 5.4.2.1). The data shown in figure 18 represents 69% of the 29 subcategories in the dataset, accounting for approximately 95% of all coded utterances in the corpus.

The most frequent subcategory in this corpus is 'promise action' with 152 occurrences. This finding is surprising given the moderate significance of this category in the dataset (cf. section 5.4.3.1). However, it illustrates Johnson's strategy of committing to decisive action by indicating that the government is aware of an issue, is treating it with the appropriate level of seriousness and is implementing effective solutions. The outcome may be to address the problem itself on the one hand, and to reassure the public on the other. Demonstrating that the government is not indifferent to their situation may cause individuals to feel acknowledged and less isolated, even amid spatial isolation.

Figure 18: Distribution of the 20 most frequent speech act subcategories in the JPanC20; sorted by absolute frequency; categories coded by colour: red: expressives, green: assertives, orange: commissives, yellow: directives, blue: declaratives

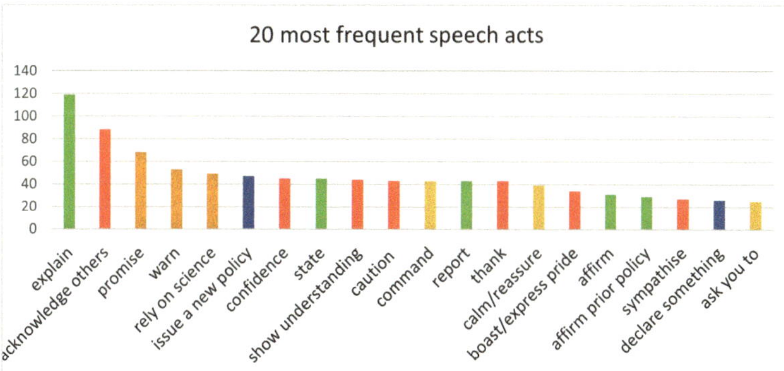

Furthermore, the impression of being committed to addressing the issue at hand may constitute the second major objective of the securitizing move, alongside warning of a threat. It reinforces the portrayal of the prime minister as a capable and powerful politician. By publicly promising action, Johnson and his government signal accountability, strengthening the perception of their commitment to resolving the crisis. This reinforces the idea that the leadership is determined and capable of addressing the problem, which enhances trust in the government's plans and policies. Lastly, these promised actions frequently outline plans that rely on public support or compliance, for example by adhering to restrictions. By proclaiming such commitments, Johnson may encourage citizens to support government initiatives, implying that collective action will lead to the desired positive outcomes.

The **second most frequent subcategory**, with 131 instances, is the expressive 'express gratitude'. These utterances demonstrate the emphasis on cooperation in Johnson's crisis communication, as he explicitly acknowledges the efforts of others in combating the crisis through various means. He draws attention to the contributions of various social groups, including, but not limited to, the military, politicians engaged in crisis mitigation and groups of essential workers, such as NHS staff, teachers and transport or postal workers. However, the primary addressee is the British public. Frequently thanking them for their daily sacrifices and deliberate efforts to comply with the restrictions, Johnson highlights that their behaviour is essential to fight the threat posed by the virus. He emphasises his belief that the situation requires the involvement of the entire nation and can only be addressed through collective action, thereby attempting to instil a sense of purpose as well as collective pride in the progress made. Explicitly expressing gratitude to individuals or groups in this way conveys the government's appreciation and contributes to the perception that individual contributions are valued by the nation. This, in turn, may enhance the likelihood of continued efforts. Concurrently, expressions of gratitude for the public's support in countering threats by the securitising actor acknowledge the audience's acceptance of the speaker's narrative, thereby reinforcing its perceived credibility. This may, in turn, persuade undecided or dissenting citizens to align with the prime minister's position, as it appears to be a successful and widely endorsed approach.

Gratitude exemplifies the emphasis on emotions in Johnson's approach. If all expressions of emotions in the dataset – comprising almost all expressive speech acts – are added together, this results in a total of 410 speech acts. This combined total is far greater than any of the subcategories depicted in figure 18, which illustrates the particular significance of expressing emotions in the context of the prime minister's crisis communication. It is the display of emotions, rather than an appearance of neutrality or indifference, that helps create a sense of empathy and solidarity with the public during a time marked by pervasive uncertainty and fear about health, personal safety and economic well-being. By conveying emotions, Johnson portrays himself as a humble and approachable prime minister, thereby establishing a personal connection with citizens and acknowledging their concerns and hardships. This emotional engagement plays a crucial role in fostering a sense of shared experience and reassurance, which in turn motivates the nation to contribute to the collective endeavour, even in the face of challenging and uncomfortable measures. It humanises the leader, making the communication more relatable and persuasive.

As previously outlined, explanations are the most prevalent speech act with 119 instances. They also represent the **most common subcategory of assertives**. Their role has already been elaborated on in section 5.4.6.1. However, it is noteworthy that all seven assertive subcategories are present in figure 18, i.e. all of them occur more than 18 times in the *JPanC20*. This indicates the relatively high significance of both the category and the individual subcategories. It seems that not only explanations but also reports, affirmations, statements, descriptions as well as narrating and answering speech acts represent substantial components of the prime minister's securitizing act.

The **most frequent subcategory of declaratives** is the announcement of new measures with 63 occurrences. The high occurrence of declarative speech acts during the initial phase of securitization is unexpected as they are traditionally associated with the second phase, the implementation of emergency measures. However, the data suggest that there is an overlap in phases, with the securitizing move and policy implementation occurring simultaneously. This dynamic process reflects the volatile nature of the crisis, requiring continuous adaptation to the evolving threat and public response. This can be interpreted in various ways, leading to theoretical discussions about the securitization framework. On the one hand, it may merely signify that the first and second phases of securitization overlap in practice. Furthermore, as stated in section 2.2.2, the acceptance of the speaker's narrative is evident in the passage of the proposed new bills in parliament. The consequences for the public would therefore stem from this prior acceptance by their representatives. The nine-month analysis period further explains the repeated iterations of the securitizing move, which ultimately led to the issuance of measures. This suggests that the phases do in fact overlap in practice. However, the prime minister's readiness to act without an explicit public consensus may suggest that acceptance is determined only after the initial imposition of measures countering the perceived threat, with adherence or non-adherence to these new rules serving as an indicator of acceptance. This understanding would differentiate between acceptance within the in-group – in this case the British public – and acceptance granted by the parliament as the public's representatives, representing forms of primary and secondary acceptance. This theoretical perspective invites further discussion about the specific threshold for acceptance, which likely to vary according to the particular circumstances of each case. In this case study, however, both acceptance by members of parliament and by the majority of British citizens are given, as shown by the relatively small percentage of Britons who spoke out against or dissented from the government's measures in the analysed period (cf. Vizard 2020: Table 5; Cabinet Office 2023: 1; Shepherd et al. 2023: 2).

Consequently, the prevalence of this subcategory may not be theoretically expected. Empirically, however, it is unsurprising at this early stage of the pandemic, given the government's efforts to combat the surge in infection rates and their associated negative impacts. These efforts include the implementation of novel policies and the dissemination of evolving guidelines. This subcategory also highlights Johnson's role as a government official and a member of the executive branch, thereby emphasising the authoritative component of this communication strategy.

In contrast, directives are expected in the securitizing move. As figure 18 demonstrates, all four of the **directive speech act subcategories** are present in the 20 most frequent subcategories. With 86 coded utterances, the most frequent subcategory in directives is 'request'. Being more polite and less authoritative than commands, which are at position ten in this list, they highlight Johnson's collaborative approach to mitigating the crisis. The predominant individual speech act in this category is 'calm/reassure' with 39 occurrences, followed by 'ask you to' with 25 instances. It can be observed that the former shares a similar intention with the aforementioned commissive 'promise of action' or assertive 'explain', thereby amplifying their overall impact. Their common objective is to provide comfort and reassurance to the public by indicating that the government is successfully addressing the crisis. This instils confidence that concrete and effective steps are being taken to manage the situation, thereby reducing stress and anxiety among individuals. Similarly, the speech act 'ask you to' contributes to the deliberate and methodical image of the prime minister as it evokes the notion of a government working strategically and collaboratively with the public to contain the threat. By issuing directives designed to alleviate feelings of panic and maintain social stability and the impression of deliberate action, the prime minister is providing the population with a sense of safety and control. This approach has the potential to foster a sense of unity and collective effort in overcoming the crisis, a sentiment particularly beneficial during the pandemic.

5.4.6.3 Co-occurring speech act categories

This section examines the co-occurrence of speech act categories within the same segment of the *JPanC20*, thus revealing the underlying content relations and identifying speeches characterised by a notable number of overlapping individual speech acts. This demonstrates that individual utterances can simultaneously serve multiple communicative purposes. The speaker may, for instance, address both the informational and emotional needs of the audience in a single utterance by employing assertive and expressive speech acts. Moreover, he may also combine different speech acts with the intention of enhancing the persuasive impact of his messages, thereby ensuring that they are both informative and emotionally resonant. This suggests a deliberately planned approach designed to address the public's diverse needs while persuading them to adopt a particular standpoint or behaviour. Similarly, it is possible that a particular press statement makes particularly challenging demands, necessitating an increased use of rhetorical devices. The co-occurrences highlight the inherent complexity and multifaceted nature of language, particularly in the context of crisis communication, where the ability to convey a nuanced message through speech is often crucial.

Given that the dataset comprises 1,271 individual speech acts, the **co-occurrence rate** of 15% is relatively low. Most instances involve overlapping speech acts between **expressives and assertives**, with 49 cases distributed over 28 press statements. The most frequent co-occurrence is between the subcategories 'gratitude' and 'report', which appears six times. Occurring mostly after mid-October, these instances acknowledge that the reported progress has only been possible due to cooperation between a multitude of stakeholders and the collective effort of different entities within British society. One example can be found in the 23 November statement: "This vaccine could be both affordable and easy to use and highly effective[.] We have ordered 100m doses and thanks to the work of the Vaccines Task Force we have secured more than 350m doses of potential vaccines of all kinds" (Johnson 2020ap: 1). This references the process of creating the first existing vaccine, which is described as being financed by British taxes, manufactured by a British company and ordered by the government's Vaccines Task Force (cf. ibid.). This co-occurrence thus indicates an appreciative approach focusing on achievements and progress.

Additionally, 'report' and 'pride' are observed together on four occasions, while the highly similar 'state' and 'pride' are found together three times. Both combinations build on the previous sentiment, adding the notion of being proud of the country's collaborative efforts that led to the status quo. Moreover, there are four instances of 'affirm' co-occurring with 'express confidence', which appears to be a logical pairing as the affirmation of a prior decision inherently carries the implicit assertion that it was correct or important. This finding offers additional evidence of the prime minister's conviction that his approach is the most suitable for addressing the crisis. All other combinations of expressives and assertives are found less than three times and therefore play a minor role in Johnson's communication strategy.

Expressives and commissives co-occur in 29 cases over 15 speeches. The most frequent co-occurrence is between 'express gratitude' and 'promise action', occurring together seven times. This is the highest incidence of co-occurrence between any subcategories in the entire *JPanC20*. Thanking others or acknowledging their work are typically accompanied by a reference to science, such as in the 16 October statement, in which Johnson combines the most prevalent emotion, gratitude, with a promise of action: "I am grateful to the Chief Scientific Adviser and the Chief Medical Officer for their advice on the measures I am about to set out – and on this basis I can confirm the Government judges we have met the fifth test" (Johnson 2020v: 2). By communicating in this manner, the prime minister highlights his determination to remaining guided by scientific expertise, at the same time acknowledging the value of collaboration in the crisis. Committing his government to following scientific advice and reinforcing this promise by giving joint press conferences with medical and scientific advisers, this speech is illustrative of the prime minister's loyal adherence to scientific advice in the pandemic. It further reinforces the notion that Johnson is a suitable leader in times of crisis, demonstrated by his ability to navigate the current challenges with scientific support.

The next most frequent co-occurrence is between 'sympathy/understanding' and 'promise action' with four instances. This combination highlights another facet of Johnson's communication strategy. It demonstrates his commitment to addressing the concerns and issues of citizens, thereby providing assurance of active support. In turn, this portrays him as an empathetic, caring and decisive politician. All other co-occurrences appear in a maximum of three instances.

The third-highest co-occurring category combination is **assertives and commissives**, which appear together in 28 overlapping segments. 'Promise action' is primarily combined with affirmative or explanatory speech acts, occurring six times with each. The former occur predominantly during the summer months, either affirming a willingness to adhere to scientific advice or promising to continue with an established policy. This strategy again portrays the prime minister as a reliable and deliberate politician, characteristics with the potential to reassure citizens in this period of initial relief after the first lockdown.

A second combination of 'promise action' and explanations predominantly encompasses the commissive speech acts of promising or assuring the audience of the speaker's ongoing commitment to following scientific advice. The following statement is an example of the latter: "Yesterday, on the advice of the four Chief Medical Officers, the UK's Covid alert level was raised from 3 to 4, the second most serious stage, meaning that transmission is high or rising exponentially" (Johnson 2020ad: 1). As an explanation for the change in policy, he mentions the scientific assessment of the Chief Medical Officers. This articulation of the necessity for the new regulations not only demonstrates his commitment to following the advice provided but also portrays the selected approach as the sole viable and legitimate option. It narrows the perceived range of alternatives, creating a sense of inevitability that implies that the decision is not just reasonable but also necessary.

Co-occurring directives and declaratives appear six times, taking the form of commands paired with announcements of new measures. These occasions are all related to the two lockdowns. Utterances such as "From Thursday until the start of December, you must stay at home" (Johnson 2020ak: 2) or "From this evening I must give the British people a very simple instruction – you must stay at home" (Johnson 2020i: 1) vividly illustrate this duality. In their direct manner, these statements not only announce the measures but also reinforce the necessity of compliance through explicit commands. This directness enhances the weight and seriousness of the instructions, thereby emphasising the urgency and non-negotiable nature of the demanded actions. These co-occurrences condense executive authority and the power of the office, thereby embodying the authoritative element of Johnson's crisis communication.

The remaining co-occurring categories appear at a frequency of approximately ten times or less each, with individual subcategories correlating on four occasions at most. The least frequent combination of categories is assertives and declaratives, with only ten instances in the entire *JPanC20*. This may be attributed to their divergent functions, which result in them typically being used at different stages in securitizing statements. Whereas assertive speech acts convey information, describe states of affairs or assert beliefs, declaratives are characteristically employed to make formal changes to policy in authoritative statements. Consequently, the former are used to inform the audience about the perceived threat and recent developments or explain the rationale behind a policy, which typically appears at the beginning of the securitizing act. The latter constitute the result of these statements or explanations, signalling the shift from explanation to action. Combining them in close proximity may weaken the impact of either one, as assertives are designed to build credibility and declaratives aim to exert authority. Therefore, Johnson may be deliberately separating them to emphasise the transition from informing to acting.

The **statements containing the most co-occurrences** are the 24 May statement (cf. Johnson 2020q) with 11 instances and the 17 July (cf. Johnson 2020z) and 2 December statements (cf. Johnson 2020at) with eight each. All other press statements exhibit a lower frequency of speech acts pairings, with a median value of three co-occurrences per statement across the entire dataset.

The May statement commences with Johnson addressing the rumours around the Cummings scandal, which has already been discussed in section 5.4.2.7. This highly publicised controversy during the COVID-19 pandemic involved a possible lockdown rule violation by Dominic Cummings, who was then Chief Adviser to Prime Minister Boris Johnson. This statement is therefore situated within a context of increasing frustration on the part of the public, the erosion of public trust (cf. Davies et al. 2021: 4) and growing demands for consequences, which Johnson seeks to address through the statement. The high frequency of co-occurring speech acts in this speech may signal the prime minister's intensified yet unsuccessful effort to convince the nation of his narrative.

Additionally, he outlines the next steps in lifting the lockdown, in particular the phase of reopening schools, which was an explicit priority for the government (cf. Johnson 2020q: 2). Explicitly highlighting the significance of the moment for pupils, parents and teachers alike and emphasising his relief at the easing of restrictions, this press statement includes a high number of directives in the form of commands, combined with declarative announcements or commissive warnings. They reflect tentative optimism in a phase of early yet unstable progress. In contrast, assertives are mostly paired with expressions of sympathy for the hardship children have undergone or gratitude for the schools' preparations. The high rate of co-occurrences thus illustrates Johnson's cautious but carefully optimistic approach in reopening schools, which may be interpreted as attempt to steer the attention of the audience toward a success delivered by the government and to portray himself as empathetic leader. Considering the circumstances, this attempt can be categorised as futile, considering the stark decrease in public trust from this moment on (cf. Davies et al. 2021: 6).

The two press statements with the second-highest rate of co-occurrences each contain eight co-occurring speech acts. During his 17 July speech (cf. Johnson 2020z), the prime minister praises the nation for the low incidence numbers and reports on the few regions showing differing developments. Subsequently, he details preparations for the expected autumn and winter surges, including increased testing capacity and the planned vaccination programmes. A defining feature of this statement is its combination of expressing caution and promising action, particularly regarding vaccine and testing preparations aimed at countering the projected rise in infection rates in the second half of the year. The second press statement with eight co-occurrences is chronologically the last in the dataset (cf. Johnson 2020at). It announces the availability of the first vaccine, a British product, and conveys the author's cautious satisfaction regarding the accomplishment of this self-imposed milestone. This announcement sees four cases of co-occurring assertives and commissives, two of which are explanations and promises of action, with one instance of 'warn' and one of 'rely on science'. These findings demonstrate that (expected) variations in infection rates – whether increasing or decreasing – result in an elevated rate of co-occurring speech acts. However, the introduction of the most stringent restrictions does not cause the greatest number of co-occurrences. This may be due to the prime minister's attempt to communicate with unambiguous clarity in these cases to prevent confusion.

5.4.6.4 Distribution of speech act categories across speech segments

The different sections of the speeches in this corpus exhibit a distinct pattern of speech act categories. Figure 19 provides an overview of their distribution across the 46 speeches in the dataset.

For this chart, the length of the press statements was subjected to a process of **normalisation**. Using *MAXQDA*'s *Document Comparison Chart* tool, each text was divided into 100 segments of equal length. This enabled the qualitative comparison of vastly different statements, such as Johnson's Economy Speech (cf. Johnson 2020x) – the longest in the dataset, with 3,681 words across 292 paragraphs – and the shortest contribution, the brief transcript of his video message containing only 320 words in 15 paragraphs (cf. Johnson 2020k). By dividing all the texts into proportional segments, differences in document length are accounted for; this method ensures that shorter statements are not underrepresented and longer speeches do not disproportionately dominate the analysis. At the same time, this process distorts the scale of the individual speech acts, as a single segment in this dataset can contain between three and 37 words. This results in a distribution of categories that may appear to differ from the category percentages shown in figure 2 (cf. section 5.4), but it remains statistically correct. Thus, the comparison of these normalised press statements allows the identification of meaningful patterns and distributions of speech acts across diverse contexts and document sizes.

Figure 19: Distribution of speech act categories in the different parts of the press statements in the JPanC20; y-axis: press statements arranged in chronological order; x-axis: normalised length of press statements; categories coded by colour: red: expressives, green: assertives, orange: commissives, yellow: directives, blue: declaratives; white denotes other speech acts irrelevant for this analysis; striped areas indicate the co-occurrence of categories

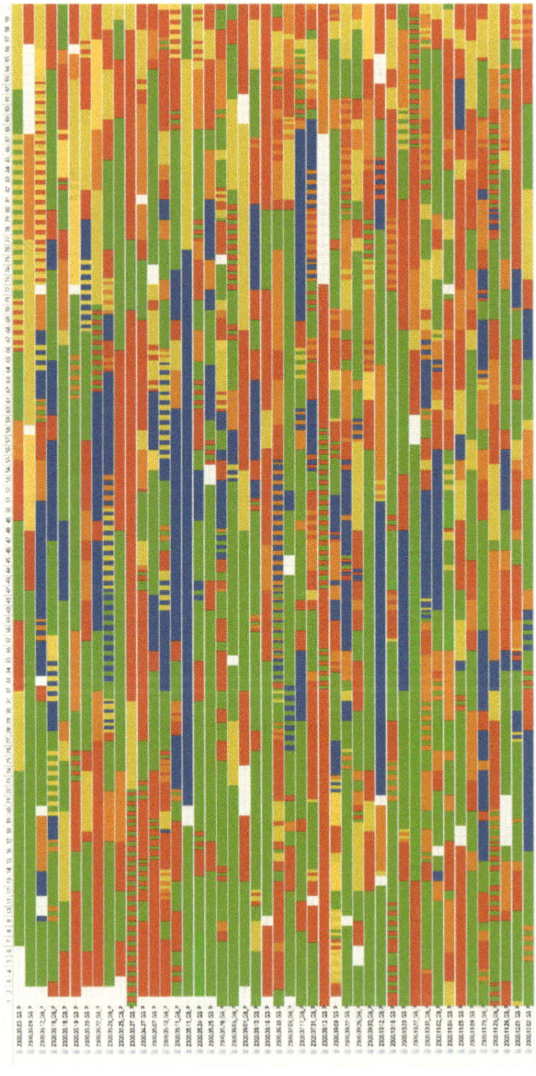

In the event of multiple codes within the same segment, the *MAXQDA* tool proportionally distributes the available space among all the codes in the paragraph. This allocation is based on the frequency with which a code has been assigned in the paragraph, rather than the length of the coded sections (cf. Verbi 2024b). Consequently, if a code is assigned twice in a paragraph and another code is assigned only once, the former code is allocated two thirds of the space while the latter code receives one third of the space. When two codes occur equally frequently in a segment, this is indicated with stripes.

In figure 19, the dominance of expressive and assertive speech acts, denoted in red and green respectively, is notable.

In the **introductory section**, assertive speech acts – indicated here in green – are most prevalent. In general, 58% of press statements are initiated with an assertive utterance. From mid-May onwards, the initial utterances are predominantly assertive, comprising primarily reporting or updating speech acts that give an account of current developments. Furthermore, a smaller number of utterances 'stating' the agenda for the press conference can be found. However, in March, April and the beginning of May, when numerical data was less readily accessible than in the second period of the dataset, a greater proportion of expressives is observed at the beginning of the statements. These are denoted in red. Mostly, they acknowledge the scientists in attendance – such as the Chief Medical Officer, or other politicians, such as Chancellor Rishi Sunak – as well as thanking segments of the public or the entire nation for their efforts (cf. Johnson 2020h: 1). Towards the end of October, two additional instances of initial expressive speech acts occur, once again acknowledging the presence of scientists and the chancellor. The two opening directive segments in November and December are due to the nature of statements in the House of Commons. Here, Johnson asks the Speaker of the House to approve his proposed policies (cf. Johnson 2020am: 1). With the exception of these infrequent outliers, Johnson's speeches typically commence with assertive speech acts that provide insight into the new figures and developments.

The **middle section of the speeches** displays a relatively high frequency of declaratives and assertives, in combination with smaller portions of commissive speech acts. Declarations, marked in blue, occur exclusively in the midsection of the corpus texts. In the majority of cases, the speech act that precedes them is an explanation (cf. Johnson 2020al: 3). This indicates that the prime minister typically elaborates on the circumstances and the associated risks – thereby facilitating a transparent understanding of the government's decision-making process – prior to the introduction of a policy or the imposition of new restrictions. About 65% of all the press statements include a declaration within this particular section, making it a characteristic feature of the corpus. The assertive speech acts in this part are predominantly explanations or affirmations, thus highlighting once again the government's objective of a transparent approach. Moreover, the aggregation of commissive speech acts in the second quarter of the speeches predominantly comprises warnings for the period between October and December. This may be attributed to the second lockdown, which began on 5 November. With utterances such as "Otherwise we face a bleak and an uncertain future of steadily rising infections and admissions until as I say the capacity of the NHS is breached" (Johnson 2020am: 1), the prime minister tries to encourage compliance with the restrictions, citing the danger to the country's health system as his main argument. A smaller number of directives can be observed in the second quarter of the press statements, otherwise these mostly occur in the last part of the statements.

While the third quarter sees a relatively equal distribution over all five categories, the **concluding section**, i.e. the final quarter, predominantly comprises assertives and directives. The latter mostly consist of reassuring and motivating statements, occasionally accompanied by orders or advice (cf. Johnson 2020ah: 3). In instances where the concluding utterance is a directive, it is predominantly either instructive or motivating and employs established slogans, such as "Stay at home, protect the NHS, and save lives" (Johnson 2020k: 1). Expressives occur with comparable frequency in the final quarter of the dataset and typically manifest as expressions of praise or confidence, or instances of gratitude (cf. Johnson 2020k: 1). The confident utterances predominantly emphasise trust in the efficacy of the government's policies, which will ultimately lead to a triumph over the virus (cf. Johnson 2020ah: 3). Gratitude is directed towards multiple contributing groups, in particular the public for their "fantastic national effort" (Johnson 2020af: 2). The prime minister may be employing this method of concluding press conferences to encourage praised groups or citizens to maintain compliance, demonstrating that their behaviour is explicitly valued by the government and the first beneficial effects are becoming apparent.

Approximately 50% of corpus elements **conclude with** an expressive speech act, often occurring in the vicinity of directives and, to a lesser extent, in combination with commissives or assertives. In this particular position, instances of confidence are often observed, frequently articulating the belief that the nation will overcome its challenges through collective action: "we will beat it together[,] we will come through this all the faster[,] and the United Kingdom will emerge stronger than ever before" (Johnson 2020l: 4). Expressions of gratitude are relatively infrequent as concluding sentiments and are primarily associated with scientific advancements, such as the announcement of successful vaccine trials. In these cases, scientists and volunteers receive particular recognition (cf. Johnson 2020at: 3). The most common concluding utterance, however, is the acknowledgement of others. On the 13 occasions where experts are present and continue with their contribution after Johnson's speech, for example at the 28 May press conference (cf. Johnson 2020s), the prime minister acknowledges them before handing over the microphone.

A further 32% of press statements end in directive speech acts. At the beginning of March, their tone is exclusively reassuring, indicating that the situation is under control (cf. Johnson 2020a: 1). However, from the evening of 23 March onwards, with the announcement of the first lockdown, the tenor of these messages shifts. They become both instructive and imploring in nature, reiterating simple behavioural guidance, either in the form of specific actions, such as handwashing, or through the use of designated slogans. One example for this is the 24 May statement: "we must remember the basics. Wash our hands, keep social distance, isolate if you have symptoms – and get a test. We (...) will beat it all the faster if we stay alert, control the virus and save lives" (2020b: 3). Johnson therefore attempts to increase the impact of his key message by concluding with a succinct and memorable slogan that citizens can easily keep in mind.

Assertives and commissives are relatively uncommon in concluding speech acts. The six instances of assertives at the end of a speech are all affirming speech acts, articulating the prime minister's conviction that the government's policies are effective and sufficient. He reiterates that these policies will enable the country to overcome the current crisis and defeat the virus. A total of three concluding commissives are found in the corpus, consisting of two warnings to stay alert in July – when low numbers were prevalent – as well as one promise "to do everything in our power" (Johnson 2020ae: 4) to overcome this challenge at the UN General Assembly in September. More typically, he utilises commissive acts in the central sections of speeches, where he is able to contextualise them with explanations about their reasons, scope and timing. The concluding remarks of his speech at the United Nations align with his overarching objective, namely to encourage other political leaders to participate in a collaborative effort against the pandemic by setting an example for other nations to follow. In contrast, the two warnings serve as the key messages in his July speeches, which were delivered at a time when public complacency could have had potentially devastating effects on the government's strategy. In order to encourage greater public awareness and vigilance, he reiterates the warning as his concluding message in both instances.

The most frequent occurrence of assertives is therefore in the initial position, especially in the period from March until July, where they are the most prevalent speech act in this particular part of the press statements. Over the length of the statements, the occurrence of assertives gradually declines, becoming sporadic in the final quarter. When positioned in the first section of press statements, assertive speech acts mostly comprise updates and reports of new developments. In the middle part, they are predominantly explanations. The inverse distribution is observed in the case of directives. Whereas they occur only very sparsely in the first half of press statements, their frequency increases significantly in the second part. Another trend emerges when the corpus elements are examined over the course of the analysed period. While the concluding directives in March are predominantly reassuring, they become more instructive and advisory in the following months. Expressives are a frequent occurrence throughout press statements in the examined time, which demonstrates Johnson's strategic use of emotive communication. When occurring at the end of a speech, they typically take the form of an expression of confidence or the acknowledgement of an expert, who then continues in the role of a speaker. The occurrence of commissive utterances is relatively infrequent within the dataset, with the majority of instances observed in the third quarter of speeches. Additionally, these expressions tend to be more prevalent in the autumn statements, where they caution against complacency and promise the relaxation of restrictions. The smallest category, declaratives, exclusively appears in the middle section of statements. The preceding speech acts typically prepare for the announcement with supporting arguments, while the subsequent ones provide an explanation or express hope that the restrictions will not remain in place for an excessive amount of time. Johnson typically concludes his speeches with a catchphrase or key thought that is both concise and memorable, allowing citizens to easily recall his main message and comply with the current set of regulations.

6 Speech Acts in the Securitizing Move

The present study is guided by the two research questions posed in section 4.2. The first of them asks about the specific speech acts employed by a securitizing actor during a securitizing move, whereas the second focuses on the prototypical structure of speech acts in the securitizing speeches delivered by British Prime Minister Boris Johnson during the COVID-19 pandemic.

In an attempted answer to the first question, section 6.1 begins with five tables of speech acts used by the British prime minister to construct and legitimise emergency measures. These are sorted according to Searle's categories, on the basis of the analysis findings from sections 5.4.1 to 5.4.6.4. Subsequently, the second research question regarding a potential prototypical structure of speech act categories in the securitizing move is addressed in section 6.2. Building on the results of the speech act category frequencies over the length of press statements in the *JPanC20* as well as their distinctive patterns in the individual communicative units (cf. section 5.4.6), a tentative model of a prototypical press statement is generated.

6.1 Mapping speech acts in the securitizing move

The first research question addresses the **individual speech acts** employed during the securitizing move by a securitizing actor. To answer this, a case study examined Boris Johnson's speech acts during the first phase of securitization in the COVID-19 pandemic (cf. chapter 5). This study is based on the *JPanC20*, consisting of 46 official press statements that were pragmatically coded for speech acts according to Searle's typology (cf. section 2.1.6). The meta-analysis in section 5.4.6 provides a detailed overview of their idiosyncrasies, whereas this section presents the relevant findings in form of a comprehensive list. Consistent with the analysis structure, the individual speech acts are sorted into categories and subcategories that display inherent interdependences. This approach allows for a detailed outline of their distribution, shedding light on their relative significance and discursive functions within the context of the British government's COVID-19 communication. The combined list of all individual speech acts sorted by frequency can be found in the appendix (cf. figure A2).

In contrast, tables 4 to 8 present a systematic overview of all 49 speech acts found in the dataset, arranged in categories. Once again, they are sorted based on absolute frequency of subcategories in the dataset. Table 4 includes all expressive speech acts present in the *JPanC20*.

Table 4: List of expressive speech act subcategories and their respective speech acts in the JPanC20; sorted by subcategory frequency

EXPRESSIVES			
Subcategory	**Speech act**	**Absolute**	**Sum**
Gratitude			**131**
	acknowledge others	88	
	thank	43	
Sympathy			**87**
	show understanding	44	
	sympathise	27	
	express regret	11	
	apologise	5	
Pride			**64**
	boast/express pride	34	
	praise others	18	
	praise himself / government	12	
Confidence			**45**
	express confidence	45	
Caution			**43**
	express caution	43	

Anger			**14**
	express anger	14	
Hope			**11**
	express hope	11	
Hedging/deflecting			**10**
	hedging/deflecting	10	
Relief			**7**
	express relief	7	
Grief			**5**
	express grief	5	
Personal experience			**4**
	personal experience	4	
Impatience			**3**
	express impatience	3	

The prevalence of expressives in the dataset underscores the fundamental role of emotions in Johnson's rhetoric during the securitizing move. In total, there are 410 utterances expressing emotions. This exceptionally high number demonstrates their significant role in Johnson's communication, highlighting their multifunctionality in conveying the complex emotional dynamics of the pandemic. In particular, the subcategory '**gratitude**' emerges as a prominent theme (cf. sections 5.4.1.1 and 5.4.6.2). These utterances represent an essential element in the prime minister's statements, as they underscore his acknowledgement of the contributions of specific groups and the general public in mitigating the threat posed by the virus. Emphasising his gratitude, he recognises their efforts and sacrifices, affirming their necessity and value for the nation. This approach not only motivates the public to cooperate further but also reinforces the perception that their efforts are highly appreciated and regarded as integral to overcoming the crisis. In doing so, it fosters a sense of collective pride in the progress made and a shared sense of purpose for Britons. Concurrently, he establishes a personal connection with the public, cultivating his image as an approachable and empathic politician.

The second most frequent subcategory, 'sympathy' (87 occurrences), primarily encompasses understanding and sympathising speech acts regarding the difficulties experienced by citizens due to the consequences of the virus and the resulting restrictions. This again contributes to a positive and empathetic image. Pride constitutes another frequent motif in the dataset, a phenomenon that may be expected of a prime minister to a certain extent. In particular, Johnson emphasises that Great Britain has responded better than other European countries to the challenges and stresses the country's success, thus attempting to motivate citizens and highlight his government's achievements. There are slightly more utterances praising others than lauding the government or himself, which suggests a deliberate effort to balance self-promotion with acknowledgement of others. This approach is designed to increase morale and foster resilience, while simultaneously reassuring the audience and affirming the government's competent and proactive management of the crisis, which can be considered crucial elements in establishing public trust and confidence. Moreover, the speech acts 'confidence' and 'caution' – with 45 and 43 speech acts respectively – contributes to this impression of balance in the dataset. They project optimism and control while acknowledging the ongoing risks and uncertainties inherent in the crisis. Each represents a singular yet significant individual speech act, illustrating the government's strategy of tentative optimism and conditional confidence in its own policies. Additionally, the speech act 'personal experience', with only four occurrences – the penultimate subcategory in table 4 – is surprisingly irrelevant for Johnson's communication. Considering the importance of sympathetic utterances, not addressing his own infection may reflect a deliberate choice to cultivate an image of competent and resilient leadership, as opposed to appearing weak or vulnerable.

It is noteworthy that the four most frequent subcategories correspond to **positive emotions**. In contrast, more negative or precautionary sentiments are associated with less frequent subcategories, such as 'anger', 'grief' or 'impatience'. They occur under specific circumstances and are not characteristic of the corpus, suggesting that such expressions are reserved for moments requiring explicit acknowledgement of loss or hardship, rather than being central to the overall communicative strategy. In general, Johnson's approach appears optimistic, with an emphasis on fostering resilience and unity among the audience through positive emotional appeals. This strategy aligns with the overarching objectives of maintaining public morale and ensuring compliance during a period of uncertainty. By predominantly framing the crisis through a positive and forward-looking lens, the prime minister suggests a narrative of collective strength and progress towards overcoming the challenges.

In conjunction with assertive speech acts, such as explanations that provide rational justifications, expressives contribute to a balanced approach combining logical reasoning with emotional engagement. This strategy aims to strengthen public trust in governmental leadership, encourage collective action and enhance the acceptance of challenging measures. Assertives are illustrated in table 5.

Table 5: List of assertive speech act subcategories and their respective speech acts in the JPanC20; sorted by subcategory frequency

ASSERTIVES			
Subcategory	**Speech act**	**Absolute**	**Sum**
Explain			**119**
	explain	119	
Report			**81**
	report	43	
	update	23	
	give examples	15	
Affirm			**60**
	affirm	31	
	affirm prior policy	29	
State			**45**
	state	45	
Narrate			**20**
	narrate	20	
Describe			**20**
	describe	20	
Answer			**19**
	answer	19	

Assertives are generally characterised by their neutral and informative stance, which is especially prevalent in the respective initial positions in the examined press statements. Johnson uses them to inform the public of recent developments and to manage expectations for the future. By presenting factual data, referencing figures and contextualising information in accessible terms, in particular with the subcategories 'report', 'state' and 'describe', Johnson positions himself as a capable and rational leader. His approach not only educates the public but also offers reassurance by portraying the government as competent and well-advised. The use of scientific advice – illustrated through figures, graphs and the presence of scientists at press conferences – instils confidence and potentially reduces dissent or criticism by framing policies as fact-based and scientifically grounded, thereby fostering a perception of unquestionable truths. Additionally, he attempts to direct public attention and assert authority while subtly guiding the national discourse.

This category has less speech act variety than expressives, however, the individual speech acts tend to occur more often. The most frequent one, '**explain**', has already been discussed above (cf. sections 5.4.2.1 and 5.4.6.1). It fulfils three principal tasks within the securitizing move. First, it describes the nature and extent of the threat. Next, it provides transparency on the rationale behind policy decisions and, lastly, it clarifies specific regulations and the corresponding behavioural expectations for citizens. The pivotal role of explanations in Johnson's communication suggests a fundamental conceptual function for the securitizing move in general. As the success of securitization depends on the **persuasiveness** of the narrative of being threatened, the securitizing actor may predominantly rely on explanations to articulate their perception, thus bridging the gap between the claim of an existential threat and the audience's willingness to consent to extraordinary measures. By offering logical, factual or contextual reasoning alongside contextual information or detailed insights into the decision-making process, explanatory speech acts contribute to the plausibility of the speaker's narrative. Thus, by facilitating the framing of the threat in a manner that resonates with the audience's cultural, social or historical context, they seek to make it more comprehensible and relatable to the audience's reality.

Furthermore, explanations are employed to elaborate on the proposed countermeasures and the mechanisms through which these will either resolve or at least mitigate the threat. These speech acts facilitate the acceptance of the proposed extraordinary measures by offering a detailed rationale for their immediate implementation, ensuring that public perception aligns with the speaker's assessment of their necessity and effectiveness. Consequently, explanations operate as a discursive instrument to establish resonance and legitimacy within the securitizing discourse. At the same time, the securitizing actor utilises explanations to inform the public of the conduct expected of them. This sets an expectation of compliance while reassuring citizens that their actions contribute to addressing the crisis, thereby instilling a sense of agency and collective responsibility. As these three types of explanations are likely to be present in all securitizing moves, explanatory speech acts may play the most crucial role in the initial phase of securitization, particularly in successful securitization attempts.

In the analysed securitizing move, the frequency of this particular speech act may have been amplified by the nature of the threat as a **public health emergency**. This may have prompted more proactive and detailed explanatory utterances, given that the general public is unlikely to be familiar with scientific terminology and the complex implications of concepts such as infection rates or airborne transmission mechanisms. Acting as an intermediary between the scientific community and the public, the prime minister employs explanatory speech acts to convey the gravity of the situation and justify the implementation of his proposed measures.

The second most frequent subcategory, '**report**', comparable in size to the second most frequent expressive subcategory (cf. table 4), encompasses individual acts such as reporting data, providing updates and giving examples. These reinforce the perception of the government as a reliable source of information, which is essential for managing public understanding and expectations during a crisis. This, in turn, has the potential to reduce the number of critical comments targeting the government as well as instances of non-compliance. In contrast, the subcategory '**affirm**' focuses on reiterating or reinforcing previously stated positions, policies or facts, thereby contributing to consistency and credibility, and maintaining a narrative of progress and success. In particular, affirmations supporting prior policies (29 occurrences) highlight the government's efforts to validate its decisions and uphold existing policies regardless of recent developments. Johnson's explicit commitment to executing his original strategy and established priorities once again reinforces his image as a foresighted and reliable leader, even in the face of challenges. This not only demonstrates his strategic capabilities but also provides reassurance to the public.

The less frequent speech acts '**narrate**' and '**describe**', with 20 occurrences each, reflect the secondary yet still relevant role of storytelling and descriptive elaboration in Johnson's securitizing move. They provide additional layers of engagement, detail and context, complementing the more dominant categories. Although less prevalent within this category and deviating from the predominantly neutral and informative tone, narrating utterances play a significant role by contributing evocative language and vivid imagery. This enhances the memorability of the prime minister's statements and engages the audience's emotions and imagination, thus creating a more persuasive narrative. This dual effect makes Johnson's message more impactful and relatable.

Assertive speech acts are thus employed to balance transparency, authority and reassurance. They aim to achieve stability and control, while also shaping the discourse in a way that legitimises government actions and minimises opposition. By combining factual clarity and contextual information with narrative elements, Johnson attempts to help the British public navigate the uncertainty and fear of the pandemic. However, commissive speech acts fulfil a different objective.

Table 6: List of commissive speech act subcategories and their respective speech acts in the JPanC20; sorted by subcategory frequency

COMMISSIVES			
Subcategory	**Speech act**	**Absolute**	**Sum**
Promise action			**152**
	promise	68	
	rely on science	49	
	commit himself to do sth	21	
	imply	11	
	vow	2	
	offer	1	
Warn			**53**
	warn	53	
Threaten			**1**
	threaten	1	

As shown in table 6, this category is comprised of three subcategories, only one of which encompasses several individual speech acts. Overall, this category is less prevalent in the dataset, yet it contains two key components of a securitizing move. In reverse order of frequency, but following the logic of the securitization framework, these are the subcategories 'warn' and 'promise of action'. Representing 25% of all commissive speech acts, **warnings** are the fourth most frequent individual speech act in the dataset (cf. figure 17). Within securitization, they are strategically employed to emphasise the severity of the threat and to delineate the potential consequences of inaction. In the *JPanC20*, warnings are not only evident at the outset of the crisis – when the nature of the existential threat is initially articulated – but also appear on later occasions to highlight risks such as the emergence of new virus variants or non-compliance with restrictions. By making these risks more tangible, warnings play a critical role in justifying proposed extraordinary measures. Concurrently, they underscore the urgency of collective action and position the government as the guardian of public well-being, while also framing individual compliance with the restrictions as a key element of the collective response. This dual function strengthens the securitizing move by fostering public trust in government decisions and encouraging adherence to directives, thereby evoking a notion of shared responsibility.

However, warnings are not the prevailing form of commissive utterances within the dataset. Instead, the subcategory 'promise of action' occurs more frequently, which suggests that the phase of the securitizing move that is characterised by warnings, may have been relatively brief. This may be due to the abrupt onset of the crisis trajectory or the British government's initial reluctance to securitize it, which may have led to a greater focus on explanations. Alternatively, this finding may indicate that Johnson prioritised a proactive communication strategy, focusing on the government's capacity to address the crisis effectively.

By emphasising **promises of action**, Johnson reinforces the image of a capable government proactively managing the pandemic, thus facilitating public confidence in his leadership. Within the framework of securitization, this type of speech act presents decisive emergency measures as necessary and vital responses by the government. Their significance within this case study reinforces the narrative that the proposed policies are indispensable, thereby positioning the administration as a key actor in safeguarding citizens. Through his promises, Johnson attempts to address concerns and demonstrate a strong dedication to mitigating the threat. Predominantly, these promises emphasise institutional rather than personal commitments in the dataset, which underscores the official responsibility and capacity of the government to manage the situation effectively, once again reinforcing the image of a competent administration capable of navigating the complex challenges posed by the pandemic.

Johnson's emphasis on **scientific input** constitutes a core element within this subcategory, as he assures the public that his decisions are guided by science. The frequent presence of advisers at press conferences, alongside the use of statistics and medical data, reinforces the perception that the government's actions are informed by expert knowledge. This, in turn, not only enhances public trust in the government's measures but also presents policy decisions as objectively necessary rather than politically motivated, therefore positioning them beyond reasonable criticism. Thus, promises of action reinforce the securitizing move by demonstrating the government's ability to act decisively while also underscoring its commitment to addressing the threat, for which it requires public compliance.

The **interplay between warnings and promises** holds particular significance in the context of securitization. The former serve to heighten the perceived severity of the threat, thus justifying the necessity of the proposed measures and fostering a sense of urgency. Conversely, promises provide a roadmap for countering the perceived threat by outlining specific actions the government will take, thereby offering stability and managing expectations. Together, these commissive speech acts align public perception with the government's narrative, simultaneously facilitating acceptance of the securitizing move and the extraordinary measures it demands. Moreover, these speech acts appeal on both an emotional and a rational level. Warnings invoke caution and vigilance, emphasising the seriousness of the threat. Promises, by contrast, convey determination, commitment and reassurance, thereby fostering trust in the government's ability to manage the crisis. This dual approach ensures the resonance of Johnson's communication with a broad audience, addressing both emotional concerns and the need for rational justification of government actions. In combination, Johnson not only strengthens his securitizing move but also reinforces his image as a rational, empathetic and authoritative figure guiding the nation through an existential crisis.

Directive utterances are another significant part of this guidance. Table 7 illustrates their distribution.

Directives are subdivided into two larger and two smaller subcategories. These differ in their instructive intensity, ranging from the encouraging 'motivate' to 'advise', 'request' and, ultimately, the authoritative 'command'. Their distribution reflects a key objective of Johnson's crisis communication: to provide clear instructions and promote collective responsibility while avoiding an overtly authoritarian tone.

Table 7: List of directive speech act subcategories and their respective speech acts in the JPanC20; sorted by subcategory frequency

DIRECTIVES				
Subcategory	**Speech act**		**Absolute**	**Sum**
Request				**86**
	calm/reassure		39	
	ask you to		25	
	implore		14	
	request		8	
Command				**58**
	command		43	
		you/we must	33	
		order	7	
		command	3	
	instruct		14	
	prohibit		1	
Advise				**18**
	advise		18	
Motivate				**17**
	motivate		17	

The most frequent subcategory, 'request', mostly involves asking for cooperation or specific actions, encouraging public participation in efforts to mitigate the crisis. Commands typically highlight the necessity of following recently introduced rules, often using the phrase 'you/we must' to underscore the importance of compliance. In contrast, the negation 'you must+not' is uncommon. Therefore, directive speech acts exemplify Johnson's attempt to **set behavioural expectations while avoiding overly restrictive language**. Instead, he instructs British citizens to adhere to recently introduced regulations while promoting their active participation in the national effort to combat the virus. He thus establishes clear expectations for citizens' actions while simultaneously alleviating anxiety and panic. These utterances increase the likelihood of public compliance and collaboration as they are designed to regulate behaviour in addition to fostering a sentiment of collective strength and resilience.

Directives contribute to the securitizing move by linking the threat to actionable steps for the audience. This is evident in various forms within the corpus. Commands present compliance with new rules as crucial for the survival and well-being of the nation, emphasising the severity of the threat and the necessity of collective action. These speech acts are particularly contingent upon the position of the speaker to unfold their illocutionary force. The realisation of this potential requires the audience's prior acceptance of the proposed measures. Furthermore, requests in the form of reassuring utterances mitigate public anxiety while encouraging cooperation, thereby facilitating public trust and adherence to established measures. Similarly, advisory speech acts provide clear and practical guidance, ensuring that the public comprehends the ramifications of the measures. Lastly, motivational utterances, often invoking role models such as Captain Sir Thomas Moore, highlight the collective effort required to overcome the crisis. Moreover, the prime minister's directives employ simple and easily comprehensible language, ensuring that his messages are accessible to the widest possible audience. This linguistic simplicity of Johnson's directive statements not only facilitates understanding but also enhances the likelihood of compliance.

Table 8 summarises the occurrence of declarative speech acts in the *JPanC20*.

Table 8: List of declarative speech act subcategories and their respective speech acts in the JPanC20; sorted by subcategory frequency

DECLARATIVES			
Subcategory	**Speech act**	**Absolute**	**Sum**
Announce measures			**63**
	issue a new policy	47	
	impose rules	16	
Declare something			**26**
	declare something	26	
Lift measures			**9**
	lift measures	9	

Declarative speech acts fulfil an important role in the dataset, although their low frequency suggests that Johnson is consciously avoiding an overtly authoritarian style of communication. A similar pattern can also be observed with directives.

These utterances often signal pivotal moments in the pandemic, such as the initiation of new phases or policy modifications, thereby redefining the definition or conditions of the threat, countermeasures and progress. By using utterances that introduce new policies, which account for over 60% of this category, Johnson translates complex and dynamic crisis developments into distinct stages that citizens can grasp, allowing them to modify their behaviour accordingly. As with directive speech acts, this simplification is essential as it enables the government to reach a significant proportion of Britons. Declaratives, therefore, function as rhetorical tools to initiate and legitimise the proposed countermeasures within the securitizing move, simultaneously marking critical junctures in the development of the situation. Furthermore, they establish authority and assert control, effectively reflecting the government's executive power.

As discussed in section 5.4.6.2, the high frequency of the subcategory 'announce measures' – encompassing the sixth most prevalent individual speech act 'issue a new policy' and the rarer 'impose rules' (cf. figure 17) – suggests a more dynamic process of securitization than previously documented. As a result, the traditional linear understanding of the three phases is challenged in favour of a concept of multiple iterations of the securitizing move. In a similar fashion, the presence of the smallest declarative subcategory can be explained by this reconceptualisation. Lifting measures, expected only in the third phase of desecuritization, may occur in the corpus under examination because of the process's repetitive structure. In order to issue novel policies and implement measures that align more closely with recent developments, it is imperative to lift the obsolete, no longer suitable rules beforehand.

This category therefore serves as a vital mechanism for government control of public behaviour. With his declarations, Johnson shapes the understanding of the evolving nature of the threat and of key turning points. By leveraging the authoritative illocutionary force inherent in these acts, the government asserts its power to define the threat and prescribe the necessary measures to address it. This direct expression of executive authority creates the foundation for public compliance, which is indispensable for the success of the securitizing move. Therefore, declarative speech acts not only reinforce the perception of governmental control and authority but also ensure that the process is anchored in clear and official communication.

6.2 Characteristic speech act patterns in the securitizing move

The subsequent section will address the second research question: What is the prototypical structure of speech acts in the securitizing speeches delivered by British Prime Minister Boris Johnson during the COVID-19 pandemic?

Section 5.4.6 describes the most frequently occurring speech acts, both at the individual speech act level and the subcategory level. This offers valuable insights into the recurrent patterns and sequences employed by the prime minister in this case study of a successful securitizing move. In conjunction with the findings from the analysis of co-occurring speech act categories, they highlight the fundamental communicative intentions and priorities of his communication strategy. Whereas the answer to the first research question required a corpus of all the press statements from the period under examination, the second research question focuses on the prototypical structure of speech acts in securitizing speeches delivered by British Prime Minister Johnson during the COVID-19 pandemic.

In order to achieve the **prototypical validity** required to answer this question, the dataset was subjected to further scrutiny. The term 'prototypical' denotes a typical example of a phenomenon, excluding outliers (cf. Cambridge Dictionary 2024b). Consequently, in order to identify a prototypical structure of speech acts in press statements during the securitizing move, corpus elements must be as structurally coherent as possible. The *JPanC20* is primarily comprised of press conferences and parliamentary statements, which represent institutionalised forms of governmental communication. In these instances, the speaker addresses the national audience directly. These settings are characterised by specific rhetorical strategies designed to inform, persuade and manage public perception, aligning with this study's focus on securitizing speech acts. While some corpus elements adopt a different format, they still serve these same objectives. Besides his video message (cf. Johnson 2020k)[1], the prime minister's two articles in newspapers (cf. Johnson

1 The deliberations about the inclusion of this corpus element can be found in chapter 5.2.3.

2020p and 2020ab) also fall into this category. Consequently, these three press statements have been evaluated and deemed acceptable.

However, a small number of corpus elements deviate from this pattern:

- the Global Vaccine Summit closing remarks (cf. Johnson 2020u), and
- the Speech to the United Nations General Assembly (cf. Johnson 2020ae).

In these two speeches, the audience is international rather than national and is limited to a specific group comprising other heads of government, as opposed to the British nation. Secondly, the communicative objective appears to be diplomatic signalling, as opposed to engaging in direct crisis management. By focusing the following analysis on prototypical instances of Johnson's securitizing speech acts, the findings will accurately reflect the communicative practices and structures most pertinent to his securitizing move. Therefore, these two press releases were excluded from the analysis addressing the second research question.

This process thus yields a coherent subcorpus comprising 44 press statements. After normalising them once again for statement length (cf. section 5.4.6.4), which ensures the comparability of the texts irrespective of their varying lengths, the predominant speech act category for each of the 100 segments was calculated with the assistance of the *Document Comparison Chart* tool in *MAXQDA* (cf. Verbi 2024b). Exporting these results into *Microsoft Excel* enabled the calculation of frequency distributions for each category across the normalised length of each press statement. The results of this process are depicted in five graphs below, showing the cumulative frequency of each category in each section of all 44 press statements.

Figure 20 illustrates the **development of expressives** across the length of the press statements.

Starting with only five occurrences of expressive speech acts in position one, the graph then shows a sharp increase, peaking at a value of 15 at position four, indicating a notable rise in expressive behaviour. Subsequently, a gradual decline extends until segment 13, where a new peak of 15 expressive speech acts is observed. The line then sees a decline with smaller fluctuations, dropping to a value below five at position 33. From this point, the overall trend reverses into a moderate rise characterised by four distinct increases until segment 65. After this period of growth, the graph declines sharply, reaching its lowest point at position 73 with only three speech acts. In the final quarter, it rises sharply, featuring three distinct peaks, each higher than the previous one. These occur at position 81 (11 speech acts), position 85 (12 speech acts) and position 90 (15 speech acts). Following a final decline to a value of ten, the graph attains its maximum value of 18 expressives at the 100th segment.

Figure 20: Frequency development of expressives across the length of press statements; subcorpus of 44 press statements from the JPanC20; x-axis: position in the press statements, normalised, trend line polynomial of degree six; y-axis: frequency of speech acts

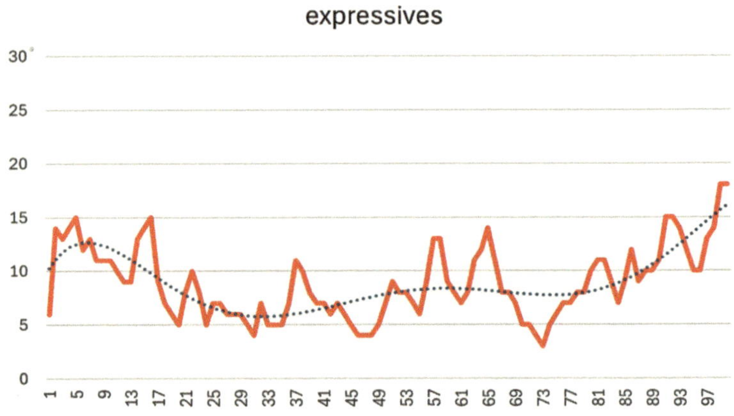

To sum up, expressives typically occur with a frequency ranging from 15 to three instances over the course of the press statement. A preliminary peak can be observed in the first quarter, followed by a decline in the second. The third quarter is characterised by a modest increase, concluding with the lowest frequency of expressive speech acts. Lastly, the final quarter exhibits a steady rise, culminating in an overall maximum of 18 speech acts. While occurring over the whole length of press statements, expressives are especially important at the beginning and the end, with a moderate significance in the third quarter. The dotted trendline highlights this wave-like dynamic.

The **development of assertive speech acts** is illustrated in figure 21.

Figure 21: Frequency development of assertives across the length of press statements; subcorpus of 44 press statements from the JPanC20; x-axis: position in the press statements, normalised, trend line polynomial of degree six; y-axis: frequency of speech acts

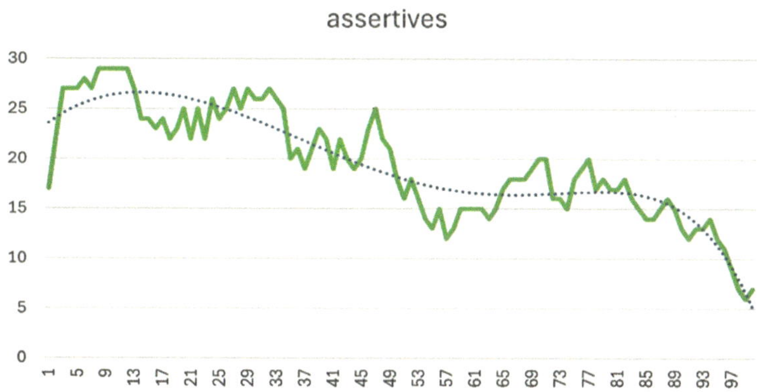

The graph begins at the notably high number of 17 assertive speech acts in the initial segment of the press statement, and this rapidly ascends to a maximum of 29 at position eight, establishing a plateau that extends until segment 11. Subsequently, it drops to 24 speech acts at position 14 before rising again to a secondary plateau of 27 between positions 27 and 32. Thereafter, a gradual moderate decline can be observed, accompanied by minor upward fluctuations, until the number of assertives decreases to 19 at position 44. A final major spike is recorded at position 47, where the number of speech acts rises to 25. In the third quarter of the segments, the graph declines steadily, reaching its first minimum of 12 assertives at segment 57, followed by a moderate resurgence with peaks up to 20 at positions 71 and 76. However, the line then drops rapidly, reaching its lowest value of six speech acts at the conclusion of the sequence.

This figure highlights the widespread distribution of assertives through almost all sections of the press statement. Initially prominent with periodic resurgences, this category generally ranges between 15 and 29 speech acts. In the final quarter, it gradually declines, followed by a sharp drop in the concluding section.

Figure 22 illustrates the **dynamic of commissive speech acts**.

Figure 22: Frequency development of commissives across the length of press statements; subcorpus of 44 press statements from the JPanC20; x-axis: position in the press statements, normalised, trend line polynomial of degree six; y-axis: frequency of speech acts

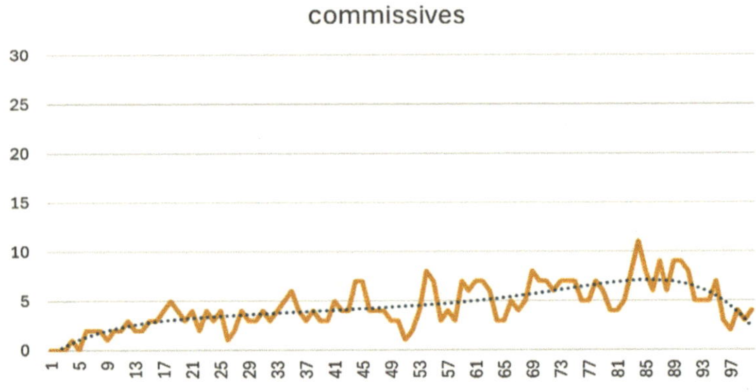

Beginning at zero in the first segment, the graph initially rises slightly, with minor peaks observed at positions 19, 35 and 45, though these generally remain low and do not exceed seven speech acts. Following a decline to one individual speech act at position 51, the graph begins a moderate ascent. This increase is characterised by minor peaks and drops, all under ten speech acts, culminating in a maximum of 11 commissives at position 84. After reaching this maximum, it descends rapidly, with a brief plateau of nine speech acts between positions 90 and 93. The graph then drops sharply to two at position 97 before concluding at a value of four.

The figure illustrates the relatively low frequency of commissive speech acts throughout the corpus, with a notable rise up to 11 speech acts in the last quarter, followed by a rapid decrease. However, except for the initial three segments of the press statement, commissives can be found in any position. This pattern suggests that commissives play a more limited but contextually concentrated role in the analysed segments.

Next, figure 23 illustrates the **distribution of directive speech acts** across the length of the press statements, as shown below in yellow.

Figure 23: Frequency development of directives across the length of press statements; subcorpus of 44 press statements from the JPanC20; x-axis: position in the press statements, normalised, trend line polynomial of degree six; y-axis: frequency of speech acts

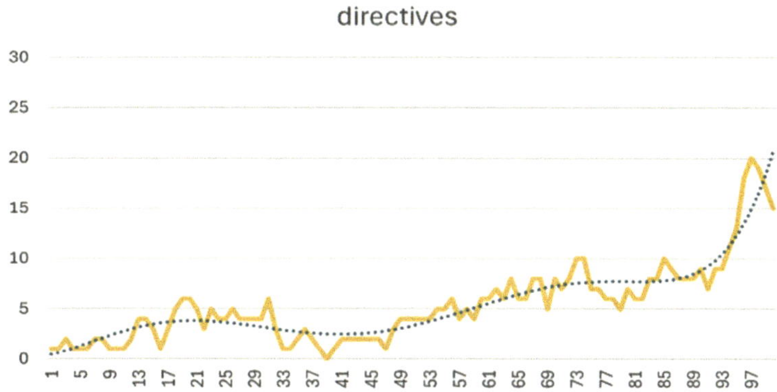

Commencing with a single directive speech act in segment one, the graph exhibits minor increments that are promptly followed by decreases until position 13, where it reaches a first small peak with four speech acts. Reverting to a single directive by segment 16, it ascends to six speech acts at position 19 but then declines. Plateauing from segment 22 with the frequency of directives remaining relatively stable at four speech acts until a spike at position 31 to the value six, the graph then drops relatively sharply to a minimum of zero at segment 39. It rises to a second plateau of two speech acts between positions 41 and 46, followed by a further gradual increase to a consistent four speech acts between segments 49 and 53. Thereafter, the curve ascends with minimal fluctuations until a small intermediate peak of ten directive speech acts at position 74. In the fourth quarter, the graph declines once again to five speech acts at segment 79, followed by an upward trend until it again reaches a peak of ten speech acts (position 85). The final downward dynamic until position 91 is immediately followed by a sudden and marked increase that exceeds the previous maximum of 11 at position 94. The increase continues to a peak of 20 directive speech acts at position 97, followed by a decrease to 15 in the final segment.

Directives thus appear to play a minor role during the first half of press statements, as evidenced by their low cumulative occurrences, with fewer than seven instances recorded at any given point. They are particularly rare in the second quarter. In the third quarter, there is a moderate increase reaching up to ten instances. The final quarter initially follows the preceding trend but then experiences a marked increase from position 94 onward, peaking at 20 instances; this is at least double the number of speech acts recorded at any point prior. It suggests that directives are employed with moderate frequency in the transition between the first and second quarters but appear infrequently in the middle section of press statements. Conversely, in the concluding sections, their occurrence increases significantly, indicating that Johnson frequently employs directives as closing remarks his speeches.

Lastly, figure 24 shows the **distribution of declaratives**.

Figure 24: Frequency development of declaratives across the length of press statements; subcorpus of 44 press statements from the JPanC20; x-axis: position in the press statements, normalised, trend line polynomial of degree six; y-axis: frequency of speech acts

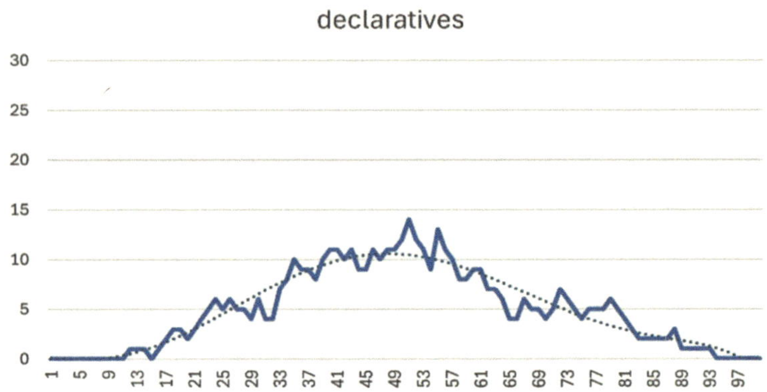

The graph shows an absence of declarative speech acts until position 12, where there is a moderate increase, reaching a peak of six speech acts at position 24. Following a brief downturn, it ascends again, reaching ten declarative speech acts in segment 35. From this point, the line exhibits minor fluctuations, arriving at a maximum of 14 speech acts at position 51. Following a second, smaller peak in segment 55 with 13 declarative speech acts, the graph gradually decreases, reaching an initial low at position 65 with a mere four speech acts. A minor increase leads to a count of seven declaratives at position 72, followed by medium-sized oscillations until position 94, where it returns to zero and maintains this value.

The distribution of declarative speech acts exhibits a gradual buildup, peaking in the middle of the document in the form of a wave, with small oscillations and sporadic fluctuations on both sides. The relatively consistent increase up to the maximum at position 51 suggests a period of heightened significance for declaratives in the central positions, subsequently giving way to a more gradual decline towards the end of the document. Notably, no declarations are observed in the initial or concluding sections.

The aggregation of these five graphs produces a comprehensive graphic that brings together the distinct developments of the different speech act categories (cf. figure 25). This enables a comparative analysis of the mean frequency dynamics of each category over the course of a press statement and the trends across the various speech act types, thereby providing a holistic understanding of their progression throughout the document.

Figure 25: Diachronic development of category frequencies across the length of press statements; subcorpus of 44 press statements from the JPanC20; x-axis: position in the press statements, normalised; y-axis: frequency of speech acts; categories coded by colour

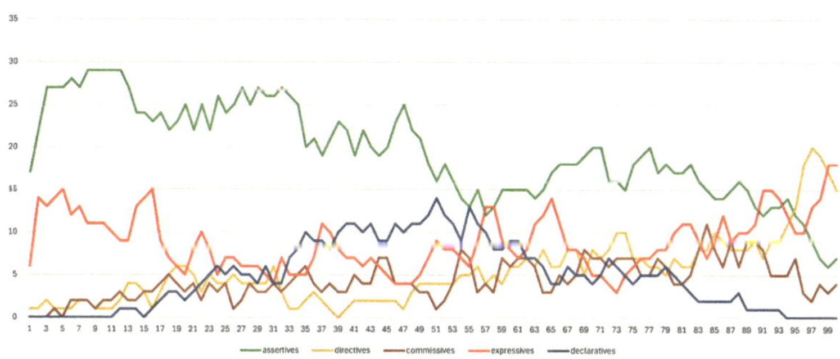

The analysis demonstrates the diachronic development of cumulative category frequencies across the length of press statements within the subcorpus. Assertives, once again marked in green, are predominant throughout the first three quarters. Initially, their numbers are nearly double those of the second most frequent category, expressives, in the first quarter. However, when expressives see a first downturn around position 17, assertives rise. Their maximum of 29 speech acts in the initial quarter is not matched by any other category in this analysis. From the second quarter onwards, a fluctuating decrease with occasional spikes can be observed for assertives. The decline becomes more pronounced towards the latter sections of the speeches, with a first local minimum at position 57 and, following a smaller section characterised by increasing numbers of assertive speech acts, a subsequent sharp drop near segment 90. This decrease coincides with an increase in declaratives in general and, to a smaller extent, with two expressive upticks. Expressives demonstrate an irregular pattern, characterised by smaller oscillations. A significant initial increase is followed by gradual decreases and fluctuations, such as the two aforementioned peaks during the descent of assertives. These speech acts, indicated in red, culminate in a pronounced rise towards the end, starting from approximately position 73 and peaking at segment 90, just below the highest category in this position, directives. They are generally the category with the second-highest number of speech acts. Directives, however, exhibit a moderate presence, which commences at a relatively low level with values below seven for over half of the press statement. Only rising from position 56 onward, this category experiences a moderate increase, characterised by fluctuations, that leads to a steep rise in the final eight segments, resulting in a maximum of 20 speech acts at position 97. In the concluding section, however, it falls under the expressive graph. In contrast, commissives exhibit a comparatively low presence throughout, with moderate increases punctuated by minor peaks, as well as a more pronounced low at position 51. Thereafter, they rise to their most notable peak of 11 speech acts in segment 84, followed by a decline below five. The commissive minimum correlates with the declarative maximum, indicating a characteristic separation of declarative and commissive utterances by Johnson. When issuing new policies, he therefore mostly refrains from committing himself or his government to specific actions. In the initial segment of the speeches, declaratives are entirely absent, which affirms their minimal significance in this portion. Beginning at position 11, concurrent with the initial assertive descent, declaratives exhibit a modest yet consistent ascent to a significant peak at position 51 with 14 speech acts. This maximum surpasses the commissive or directive trends for the majority of the statement, even approaching the development of assertives observed in the second and third quarters. Despite the fact that this figure remains below the assertives graph, it corresponds to the downward trend observed at this particular segment. The declarative numbers exhibit a decrease which mirrors their previous increase, resulting in zero instances from position 94 onwards.

This segment is evidently a pivotal point, marking a shift in the established behaviour of all categories. Position 94 signifies the commencement of directive ascent above the previous maximum of 11, along with the onset of a pronounced decline in assertives. Expressives appear to initiate their final increase slightly later, at position 96, exhibiting a certain congruence with directives. In contrast, commissives experience a final spike before undergoing a downward oscillation and dropping below seven. Consequently, the concluding section of the press statements appears to differ considerably from the other parts, placing a significant emphasis on directives and expressives and thereby signalling a rhetorical shift towards more instructive and emotionally charged communication. This may be caused by Johnson's strategy to end his statements with motivational, emotional or directive appeals. In almost all other sections, assertives are clearly predominant, and by a substantial margin. This distribution of speech acts does not resemble the one described by Schueler and Marx in their 2023 study on Dutch COVID-19 speech acts, however. All five categories manifest in distinctly different patterns than in the JPanC20, with declaratives being most prominent in the first quarter, directives and expressives occurring mostly at the beginning and assertives appearing in particular at the conclusion of the press statements. Only commissives see a slightly similar frequency distribution, albeit showing a preference for initial and concluding remarks (cf. Schueler and Marx 2023: 884f.).

However, this British finding initially appears to be incongruent with figure 2 illustrating the overall percentages of the different speech act categories (cf. section 5.4). The higher prevalence of assertives relative to expressives appears to deviate from the initial distribution of speech act categories, where expressive speech acts dominate slightly with 33%, compared to 29% for assertives. This discrepancy can be explained by the difference in the counting method employed in the various analysis stages. While the initial speech act analysis involved the absolute number of speech acts in each category, the later stage of the analysis focuses on the code length and the space it occupies. The significant difference between the two analysis results can be attributed to the tendency of expressive speech acts to use fewer words than assertive utterances (cf. figure A4 in the appendix). Thus, the detailed analysis of these graphs not only reveals the statistical tendencies and co-occurrence patterns of the five categories but also provides insights into the underlying rhetorical strategies. These findings suggest that certain speech acts are strategically clustered to serve Johnson's specific communicative goals.

Moreover, these models facilitate the identification of a pattern that characterises Boris Johnson's speeches. The following section will present the **prototypical structure** that emerges from the observed patterns. This encapsulates the functional progression and interaction of speech acts, highlighting how their positioning supports the overall rhetorical and communicative objectives.

The values for this model were calculated by identifying the predominant category for each of the 100 normalised segments. Given the relatively modest corpus size of 44 elements, an interval of three was established for determining the dominant category, thereby reducing the impact of outliers and increasing the robustness of the model. For each of the 100 segments, the predominant speech act category or categories were determined on the basis of the interval-adjusted data. Figure 26 illustrates the results, once again using colour-coding to represent the dominant speech act categories for each of the 100 segments. In cases of category overlap, striped sections indicate the coexistence of multiple dominant categories.

Figure 26: Prototypical structure of securitizing speech act categories across the length of press statements; interval of 3; subcorpus of 44 press statements from the JPanC20; x-axis: position in the press statements, normalised; categories coded by colour: red: expressives, green: assertives, yellow: directives, blue: declaratives; striped sections indicate category co-occurrence

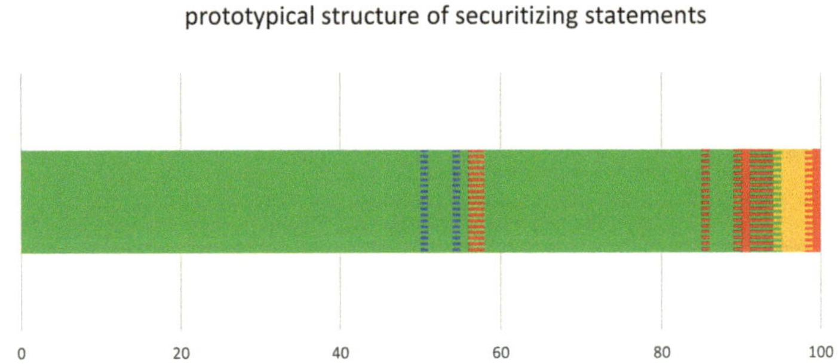

This prototypical structure of a press statement during the securitizing act by British Prime Minister Johnson during the initial phase of the COVID-19 pandemic exemplifies the distribution of speech act categories over the length of a communicative unit. The initial half is characterised by the absolute dominance of assertive speech acts. These are primarily concerned with providing factual data on the threat and information on recent developments, which is contextualised by explanations. In segments 51 and 55, the presence of ongoing assertives and two instances of declaring a policy change can be observed, thus marking a structural transition. Subsequently, in positions 57 and 58 of the model, expressive speech acts co-occur with assertives, emphasising or explaining the need for the new measures. At the same time, emotive expressions may establish an emotional connection with the audience. Assertive statements continue to dominate until segment 85, describing and explaining the implications of the new regulation. Afterwards, a notable shift in rhetoric is observed. The concluding part of the statement is initiated by the potential occurrence of expressives or assertives in positions 86 and 90 respectively, followed by a segment of expressive dominance in position 91 conveying the emotional context of the situation, such as the speaker's confidence, caution or reassurance. In the three subsequent units, a further duality of expressives and assertives is observed, prior to a transition to either directives or expressives. Four segments are predominantly directive, characteristically containing the most important rules guiding the audience's next actions and behaviours in accordance with the new policy. Segment 99 can once again contain either directives or expressives, giving way to a final expressive speech act in segment 100, which often serves to solidify the emotional and rhetorical closure of the securitizing move. Notably, commissives – coded in orange – are not visible in this model, as they do not emerge as the predominant speech act in any segment of the corpus.

While this model may not be universally observed in press statements during other successful securitizing moves, the British case of a successful COVID-19 securitizing move does adhere to this structure. Therefore, it provides a tentative framework for understanding the communicative strategies underpinning successful securitizing moves by highlighting the strategic distribution and clustering of speech act categories. It thus offers a starting point for future research in pragmatic discourse analysis in the context of securitization and crisis communication. At the same time, it invites further exploration of how variations in speech act sequences influence audience reception and the overall effectiveness of securitization efforts.

7 Conclusion and Outlook

This study examined British Prime Minister Johnson's speech acts during his securitizing move in the COVID-19 pandemic. Using methods from corpus-assisted discourse analysis, a pragmatically annotated corpus of the prime minister's press statements from 2020 was examined for common speech acts and frequent categories and subcategories in order to identify the speech acts in use and to establish characteristic distributive patterns. In light of the findings of this study, several questions and possibilities emerge that merit further attention in future research.

In order to analyse the speech acts employed by Boris Johnson in this instance of securitization, a corpus of his press statements – the *JPanC20* – was created. Serving as the foundation for this work, it has been annotated pragmatically for speech acts. This **annotated corpus** may prove useful for further research on speech acts or on different elements of Johnson's crisis communication. In light of this, the corpus has been made publicly available on the platfom Zenodo (cf. Holze 2026), thus facilitating its potential contribution to future corpus-based research in linguistics and the subfield of political linguistics. One potential avenue for utilisation would be to compare it with Johnson's rhetorical style during the later stages of the pandemic, e.g. in the desecuritization phase. A compelling research question would be to explore whether his speech acts in this phase diverge from those observed in the initial phase. Similarly, an analysis of his securitizing speech acts in Brexit-related communication – another example of a securitization attempt by the same politician – would be a valuable avenue for further investigation. This could shed light on the question of whether a pandemic differs significantly from other instances of securitization in terms of speech acts. Such findings could help establish a more robust pattern of Johnson's typical speech acts during a securitizing move.

In the *JPanC20*, **explanations** constituted the most frequent individual speech act by a significant margin. Considering that the success of securitization depends on the persuasiveness of the securitizing actor's narrative, this prominence lends support to the hypothesis that explanations are a characteristic of securitizing speech acts. Consequently, further research into other cases of securitization by different speakers is therefore necessary to test this hypothesis. However, there is a possibility that this speech act was particularly prevalent here due to the nature of the threat as a public health crisis. Since the public is likely to be unfamiliar with the scientific jargon typically used to convey information in such circumstances, they may require more detailed explanations than in other situations. The prime minister would thus serve as an intermediary between the scientific community and the public in response to the medical emergency, thereby initiating a series of explanatory speech acts. Other types of emergencies may well exhibit different characteristics. It could be argued that certain military or environmental threats, such as an invasion or flooding, would be more readily comprehensible due to their more frequent presence in our collective consciousness, either due to the extensive media coverage of such incidents, whether in journalism or fiction, or as a consequence of the frequency of such occurrences worldwide. Therefore, a comparative analysis of securitization attempts across different types of emergencies is crucial to gain a deeper understanding of the manner in which the nature of a threat influences the role of explanatory speech acts in the securitizing move.

Similarly, these findings for Boris Johnson should be compared to the rhetoric of other politicians. To ascertain the validity of this study's results in other contexts, an examination of the speech acts used by different political leaders **during the same securitizing move** is essential. As the COVID-19 pandemic was treated as a securitization situation around the globe, it presents a rare opportunity to conduct a comparative analysis of speech act patterns across countries and even continents. Initially, this could include other English-speaking countries with shared cultural characteristics, such as members of the Commonwealth. Additionally, geographical similarities could be considered, e.g. through analysing securitizing speech acts by New Zealand's prime minister Jacinda Ardern or Iceland's Katrín Jakobsdóttir as examples of other island nations. In a second step, countries with different cultural backgrounds could be considered, such as Nigeria, Jamaica and India, as representatives of nations with a shared past, or Mozambique and Brazil, as examples of nations without close cultural ties to the United Kingdom.

Alternatively, an overview of speech acts used in neighbouring European countries would contribute to the understanding of success in this particular case of securitization. Despite the use of different languages, these countries share certain geographic and cultural similarities that may be reflected in their governments' use of speech acts.

Particularly relevant in this context might be an analysis of then-chancellor Merkel's communication in Germany. Reinforced by her background as a physicist, her communication has often been characterised as pragmatic, analytic and matter-of-fact (cf. Kneuer and Wallaschek 2020: 687). In the initial phase of the pandemic, Merkel's calm and personable media presence differed notably from both her usual persona and that of other political leaders, particularly in her use of metaphors (cf. Jaworska 2021: 8). Comparing her speech acts during the securitizing move to Johnson's could therefore help determine whether the findings and proposed speech act model are applicable to such disparate rhetorical styles.

Additionally, this study identified a **high frequency of expressive speech acts** within the *JPanC20*. This might be another characteristic element of a securitizing actor's rhetoric during the securitizing move, with the speaker attempting to convey their sense of threat and concern about the well-being of a group or nation. To communicate these emotions, a variety of expressive utterances may typically be employed. It would be worthwhile to investigate whether the prevalence of expressives represents a distinctive feature of a successful securitization attempt or is merely a characteristic of Johnson's rhetorical style. In addition to Angela Merkel, who is renowned for her straightforward rhetoric, a suitable comparison could be made using the public speeches of different leaders with distinctive styles, such as those engaged in religious securitization – for example the Iranian government – or those pursuing military securitization, for example the Thai government or the government of Myanmar following the 2021 military coup (cf. Spring Research Team 2022).

Adopting an alternative perspective may prove beneficial in monitoring the success of the securitizing move from the standpoint of the audience. Their reception of the speech acts is the decisive factor in the securitization process. As the British reaction to Johnson's handling of the pandemic and many of his statements was very negative, a study that meticulously tracks the responses and spontaneous **reactions of the public** to individual speech acts could provide invaluable insight into this initial phase. However, this endeavour would appear to exceed the conventional methodologies typically employed in linguistic research, potentially requiring the input of disciplines such as media reception studies or neuroscience – particularly those subfields concerned with cognitive neuroscience or neuropsychology.

In addition, further research could benefit from the examination of the **role of the media** in the success of a securitizing move. Utilising the present *JPanC20* as a starting point, it would be interesting to analyse the speech acts and information that the media extracts from the prime minister's press conferences during this period. One potential question is whether certain speech acts are more likely to be adopted without modification. Conversely, the securitized issue could be exceptional enough to lead to a (more) standardised approach in media coverage.

These diverse ideas for further research all aim to identify overarching patterns within successful securitization attempts and assess their alignment with this study's findings. This analysis of Boris Johnson's communication during the securitizing move pertaining to the pandemic thus serves as a springboard for further linguistic investigation into speech acts that are characteristic of the initial phase of securitization and those that are particularly conducive to its success.

References

Primary Sources: JPanC20

Johnson, B. (2020a): *Prime Minister's statement on coronavirus (COVID-19): 3 March 2020*. 03.03.2020, London. Available at: https://www.gov.uk/government/speeches/pm-statement-at-coronavirus-press-conference-3-march-2020 [Accessed 9 October 2024].

Johnson, B. (2020b) *Prime Minister's statement on coronavirus (COVID-19): 9 March 2020*. 09.03.2020, London. Available at: https://www.gov.uk/government/speeches/pm-statement-on-coronavirus-9-march-2020 [Accessed 9 October 2024].

Johnson, B. (2020c) *Prime Minister's statement on coronavirus (COVID-19): 12 March 2020*. 12.03.2020, London. Available at: https://www.gov.uk/government/speeches/pm-statement-on-coronavirus-12-march-2020 [Accessed 9 October 2024].

Johnson, B. (2020d) *Prime Minister's statement on coronavirus (COVID-19): 16 March 2020*. 16.03.2020, London. Available at: https://www.gov.uk/government/speeches/pm-statement-on-coronavirus-16-march-2020 [Accessed 9 October 2024].

Johnson, B. (2020e) *Prime Minister's statement on coronavirus (COVID-19): 18 March 2020*. 18.03.2020, London. Available at: https://www.gov.uk/government/speeches/pm-statement-on-coronavirus-18-march-2020 [Accessed 9 October 2024].

Johnson, B. (2020f) *Prime Minister's statement on coronavirus (COVID-19): 19 March 2020*. 19.03.2020, London. Available at: https://www.gov.uk/government/speeches/pm-statement-on-coronavirus-19-march-2020 [Accessed 9 October 2024].

Johnson, B. (2020g) *Prime Minister's statement on coronavirus (COVID-19): 20 March 2020*. 20.03.2020, London. Available at: https://www.gov.uk/govern

ment/speeches/pm-statement-on-coronavirus-20-march-2020 [Accessed 9 October 2024].
Johnson, B. (2020h) *Prime Minister's statement on coronavirus (COVID-19): 22 March 2020*. 22.03.2020, London. Available at: https://www.gov.uk/government/speeches/pm-statement-on-coronavirus-22-march-2020 [Accessed 9 October 2024].
Johnson, B. (2020i) *Prime Minister's statement on coronavirus (COVID-19): 23 March 2020*. 23.03.2020, London. Available at: https://www.gov.uk/government/speeches/pm-address-to-the-nation-on-coronavirus-23-march-2020 [Accessed 9 October 2024].
Johnson, B. (2020j) *Prime Minister's statement on coronavirus (COVID-19): 25 March 2020*. 25.03.2020, London. Available at: https://www.gov.uk/government/speeches/pm-statement-on-coronavirus-25-march-2020 [Accessed 9 October 2024].
Johnson, B. (2020k) *PM video message on coronavirus: 27 March 2020*. 27.03.2020, London. Available at: https://www.gov.uk/government/speeches/pm-video-message-on-coronavirus-27-march-2020 [Accessed 9 October 2024].
Johnson, B. (2020l) *PM statement in Downing Street: 27 April 2020*. 27.04.2020, London. Available at: https://www.gov.uk/government/speeches/pm-statement-in-downing-street-27-april-2020 [Accessed 9 October 2024].
Johnson, B. (2020m) *Prime Minister's statement on coronavirus (COVID-19): 10 May 2020*. 10.05.2020, London. Available at: https://www.gov.uk/government/speeches/pm-address-to-the-nation-on-coronavirus-10-may-2020 [Accessed 9 October 2024].
Johnson, B. (2020n) *PM statement in the House of Commons: 11 May 2020*. 11.05.2020, London. Available at: https://www.gov.uk/government/speeches/pm-statement-in-the-house-of-commons-11-may-2020 [Accessed 9 October 2024].
Johnson, B. (2020o) *Prime Minister's statement on coronavirus (COVID-19): 11 May 2020*. Available at: 11.05.2020, London. https://www.gov.uk/government/speeches/pm-statement-on-coronavirus-11-may-2020 [Accessed 9 October 2024].
Johnson, B. (2020p) *Prime Minister's article in the Mail on Sunday: 17 May 2020*. 17.05.2020, London. Available at: https://www.gov.uk/government/speeches/prime-ministers-article-in-the-mail-on-sunday-17-may-2020 [Accessed 9 October 2024].
Johnson, B. (2020q) *Prime Minister's statement on coronavirus (COVID-19): 24 May 2020*. 24.05.2020, London. Available at: https://www.gov.uk/government

/speeches/pm-press-conference-statement-24-may-2020 [Accessed 9 October 2024].

Johnson, B. (2020r) *Prime Minister's statement on coronavirus (COVID-19): 25 May 2020*. 25.05.2020, London. Available at: https://www.gov.uk/government/speeches/pm-press-conference-statement-25-may-2020 [Accessed 9 October 2024].

Johnson, B. (2020s) *Prime Minister's statement on coronavirus (COVID-19): 28 May 2020*. 28.05.2020, London. Available at: https://www.gov.uk/government/speeches/pm-press-conference-statement-on-the-five-tests-28-may-2020 [Accessed 9 October 2024].

Johnson, B. (2020t) *Prime Minister's statement on coronavirus (COVID-19): 3 June 2020*. 03.06.2020, London. Available at: https://www.gov.uk/government/speeches/pm-statement-at-the-coronavirus-press-conference-3-june-2020 [Accessed 9 October 2024].

Johnson, B. (2020u) *PM Global Vaccine Summit closing remarks: 4 June 2020*. 04.06.2020, London. Available at: https://www.gov.uk/government/speeches/pm-global-vaccine-summit-closing-remarks-4-june-2020 [Accessed 9 October 2024].

Johnson, B. (2020v) *Prime Minister's statement on coronavirus (COVID-19): 10 June 2020*. 10.06.2020, London. Available at: www.gov.uk/government/speeches/pm-statement-at-the-coronavirus-press-conference-10-june-2020 [Accessed 9 October 2024].

Johnson, B. (2020w) *Prime Minister's statement on coronavirus (COVID-19): 16 June 2020*. 16.06.2020, London. Available at: https://www.gov.uk/government/speeches/pm-statement-at-the-coronavirus-press-conference-16-june-2020 [Accessed 9 October 2024].

Johnson, B. (2020x) *PM Economy Speech: 30 June 2020*. 30.06.2020, Dudley. Available at: https://www.gov.uk/government/speeches/pm-economy-speech-30-june-2020 [Accessed 9 October 2024].

Johnson, B. (2020y) *Prime Minister's statement on coronavirus (COVID-19): 3 July 2020*. 03.07.2020, London. Available at: https://www.gov.uk/government/speeches/prime-ministers-statement-on-coronavirus-covid-19-3-july-2020 [Accessed 9 October 2024].

Johnson, B. (2020z) *Prime Minister's statement on coronavirus (COVID-19): 17 July 2020*. 17.07.2020, London. Available at: https://www.gov.uk/government/speeches/pm-statement-on-coronavirus-17-july-2020 [Accessed 9 October 2024].

Johnson, B. (2020aa) *Prime Minister's statement on coronavirus (COVID-19): 31 July 2020*. 31.07.2020, London. Available at: https://www.gov.uk/government/speeches/prime-ministers-statement-on-coronavirus-covid-19-31-july-2020 [Accessed 9 October 2024].

Johnson, B. (2020ab) Standing side by side, we'll build back better than ever. Prime Minister Boris Johnson's article in the Belfast Telegraph newspaper. 13.08.2020. Available at: https://www.gov.uk/government/speeches/standing-side-by-side-well-build-back-better-than-ever [Accessed 9 October 2024].

Johnson, B. (2020ac) *Prime Minister's statement on coronavirus (COVID-19): 9 September 2020*. 09.09.2020, London. Available at: https://www.gov.uk/government/speeches/pm-press-conference-statement-9-september-2020 [Accessed 9 October 2024].

Johnson, B. (2020ad) *PM Commons statement on coronavirus: 22 September 2020*. 22.09.2020, London. Available at: https://www.gov.uk/government/speeches/pm-commons-statement-on-coronavirus-22-september-2020 [Accessed 9 October 2024].

Johnson, B. (2020ae) *Prime Minister's speech to United Nations General Assembly: 26 September 2020*. 26.09.2020, New York. Available at: https://www.gov.uk/government/speeches/prime-ministers-speech-to-un-general-assembly-26-september-2020 [Accessed 9 October 2024].

Johnson, B. (2020af) *Prime Minister's statement on coronavirus (COVID-19): 30 September 2020*. 30.09.2020, London. Available at: https://www.gov.uk/government/speeches/prime-ministers-statement-on-coronavirus-covid-19-30-september-2020 [Accessed 9 October 2024].

Johnson, B. (2020ag) *Prime Minister's statement on coronavirus (COVID-19): 12 October 2020*. 12.10.2020, London. Available at: https://www.gov.uk/government/speeches/prime-ministers-statement-on-coronavirus-covid-19-12-october-2020 [Accessed 9 October 2024].

Johnson, B. (2020ah) *Prime Minister's statement on coronavirus (COVID-19): 16 October 2020*. 16.10.2020, London. Available at: https://www.gov.uk/government/speeches/prime-ministers-statement-on-coronavirus-covid-19-16-october-2020 [Accessed 9 October 2024].

Johnson, B. (2020ai) *Prime Minister's statement on coronavirus (COVID-19): 20 October 2020*. 20.10.2020, London. Available at: https://www.gov.uk/government/speeches/prime-ministers-statement-on-coronavirus-covid-19-20-october-2020 [Accessed 9 October 2024].

Johnson, B. (2020aj) Prime Minister's statement on coronavirus (COVID-19): 22 October 2020. 22.10.2020, London. Available at: https://www.gov.uk/government/speeches/prime-ministers-statement-on-coronavirus-covid-19-22-october-2020 [Accessed 9 October 2024].

Johnson, B. (2020ak) *Prime Minister's statement on coronavirus (COVID-19): 31 October* 2020. 31.10.2020, London. Available at: https://www.gov.uk/government/speeches/prime-ministers-statement-on-coronavirus-covid-19-31-october-2020 [Accessed 9 October 2024].

Johnson, B. (2020al) *PM Commons statement on coronavirus: 2 November.* 02.11.2020, London. Available at: https://www.gov.uk/government/speeches/pm-commons-statement-on-coronavirus-2-november [Accessed 9 October 2024].

Johnson, B. (2020am) *Prime Minister's statement to the House of Commons on coronavirus: 4 November* 2020. 04.11.2020, London. Available at: https://www.gov.uk/government/speeches/prime-ministers-statement-to-the-house-of-commons-on-coronavirus-4-november-2020 [Accessed 9 October 2024].

Johnson, B. (2020an) *Prime Minister's statement on coronavirus (COVID-19): 5 November* 2020. 05.11.2020, London. Available at: https://www.gov.uk/government/speeches/prime-ministers-statement-on-coronavirus-covid-19-5-november-2020 [Accessed 9 October 2024].

Johnson, B. (2020ao) *Prime Minister's statement on coronavirus (COVID-19): 9 November* 2020. 09.11.2020, London. Available at: https://www.gov.uk/government/speeches/prime-ministers-statement-on-coronavirus-covid-19-9-november-2020 [Accessed 9 October 2024].

Johnson, B. (2020ap) *Prime Minister's statement on coronavirus (COVID-19): 23 November* 2020. 23.11.2020, London. Available at: https://www.gov.uk/government/speeches/prime-ministers-statement-on-coronavirus-covid-19-23-november-2020 [Accessed 9 October 2024].

Johnson, B. (2020aq) *PM statement on COVID-19 Winter Plan: 23 November* 2020. Oral Statement to Parliament. 23.11.2020, London. Available at: https://www.gov.uk/government/speeches/pm-statement-on-covid-19-winter-plan-23-november-2020 [Accessed 9 October 2024].

Johnson, B. (2020ar) *Prime Minister's statement on coronavirus (COVID-19): 26 November* 2020. 26.11.2020, London. Available at: https://www.gov.uk/government/speeches/prime-ministers-statement-on-coronavirus-covid-19-26-november-2020 [Accessed 9 October 2024].

Johnson, B. (2020as) *Prime Minister's statement to the House of Commons on coronavirus regulations: 1 December 2020*. 01.12.2020, London. Available at: https://www.gov.uk/government/speeches/prime-ministers-statement-to-the-house-of-commons-on-coronavirus-regulations-1-december-2020 [Accessed 9 October 2024].

Johnson, B. (2020at) *Prime Minister's statement on coronavirus (COVID-19): 2 December 2020*. 02.12.2020, London. Available at: https://www.gov.uk/government/speeches/prime-ministers-statement-on-coronavirus-covid-19-2-december-2020 [Accessed 9 October 2024].

Secondary Sources

Abrahamsen, R. (2005) Blair's Africa: The Politics of Securitization and Fear. *Alternatives* **30** (1), 55–80.

Abramicheva, O. (2022) Johnsonism as a Linguistic Phenomenon: Professional Discursive Personality of Boris Johnson. *International Humanitarian University Herald. Philology* **1** (53), 4–10.

Acharya, A. (2020) Responding to Covid-19. *Advances in Social Sciences Research Journal* **7** (5), 29–40.

Acheoah, J. E. (2017) Searle's Speech Act Theory: An Integrative Appraisal. *American Research Journal of English and Literature*, 1–17.

Adachi, K. (2024) The undersecuritization of COVID-19 in Japan: Voluntary behavioral change as self-defense? *Security Dialogue* **55** (3), 257–273.

Addley, E. (2020) Clap for our Carers: The very unBritish ritual that united the nation. *The Guardian*, May 28, 1. Available at: https://www.theguardian.com/society/2020/may/28/clap-for-our-carers-the-very-unbritish-ritual-that-united-the-nation. Accessed 03/03/2025.

Ädel, A. (2020) Corpus Compilation. In: Paquot, M. & Gries, S. T. (eds.) *A practical handbook of corpus linguistics*. Cham, Springer, pp. 3–24.

Adesanmi, T., Adegbite, O. & Ogazie, C. (2020) The Pandemic Discourse and Education in Africa: Insights from Selected COVID-19 Speeches. In: Motsaathebe, G. (ed.) *Education in Africa: Perspectives, opportunities and challenges*. Nova Science Publishers, New York, pp. 117–145.

Ahmed, S., Rushdi, A., Saber, A. & Ali, I. (2024) COVID-19 and Advice Speech Act: A Syntactic-Pragmatic Study. *World Journal of English Language* **14** (2), 358–365.

Ahmed, Y. (2021) Securitizing COVID-19 in the United States: Trump's Identification of China as a Threat and the Deterioration of US-Sino Relations. *Proceedings of the 2nd Political Science Students' Conference Model "Pandemics and Politics"*, 14–22.

Al Kayed, M. & Al-Ghoweri, H. (2019) A Socio-Pragmatic Study of Speech Act of Criticism in Jordanian Arabic. *European Journal of Scientific Research* **153** (1), 105–117.

AlAfnan, M. & Oshchepkova, T. (2022) A Speech Act Analysis of the United Nations Secretary-General's Opening Remarks to the General Assembly Emergency Special Session on Ukraine. *Studies in Media and Communication* **10** (2), 91.

Al-Azzawi, Q. & Ali Haleem, H. (2021) "Do you speak Corona?": Hashtags and Neologisms since the COVID-19 Pandemic Outbreak. *International Journal of Linguistics, Literature and Translation* **4** (4), 113–122.

Albert, M. (2023) Climate emergency and securitization politics: towards a climate politics of the extraordinary. *Globalizations* **20** (4), 533–547.

Alexander, R. (2020) "Die Geschehnisse des Septembers 2015": Oder: Sprachkämpfe um die Flüchtlingskrise. *APuZ* **70** (30–32), 14–17.

Alghazo, S., Zemmour, S., Al Salem, M. N. & Alrashdan, I. (2021) A cross-cultural analysis of the speech act of congratulating in Kabyle and Jordanian Arabic. *Ampersand* **8**, 100075.

Alhulaybi, A. & Hemame, B. (2023) Saudi Minister of Health's Speeches Regarding to Covid-19 Pandemic, a Study in Light of Speech Acts. *Dirasat: Human and Social Sciences* **19** (6), 538–550.

Allen, W. L., Bandola-Gill, J. & Grek, S. (2024) Next slide please: the politics of visualization during COVID-19 press briefings. *Journal of European Public Policy* **31** (3), 729–755.

Almadani, W. (2020) Agreement and Disagreement About Social Changes Regarding Saudi Women on Twitter. In: Smith, A. (ed.) *Gender Equality in Changing Times*. Palgrave Macmillan, Cham, pp. 153–180.

Almadani, W. (2021) *How Hijazi Men and Women Say "NO": A Pragmatic and Discourse Analysis Study of the Speech Act of Refusal, Gender and Culture in Saudi Arabia*. Thesis. University of Sunderland, Sunderland.

Alshmaseen, O. M., Jarrah, M. & Alghazo, S. (2023) Refusal strategies used by Jordanians and Syrian refugees in Jordan. *Kervan – International Journal of Afro-Asiatic Studies* **27**, 143–169.

Alyeksyeyeva, I. O., Chaiuk, T. A. & Galitska, E. A. (2021) Coronaspeak as Key to Coronaculture: Studying New Cultural Practices Through Neologisms. *International Journal of English Linguistics* **10** (6), 202.

Anderson, W. & Semino, E. (2020) Metaphor. In: Adolphs, S. & Knight, D. (eds.) *The Routledge handbook of English language and digital humanities*. Routledge, Abingdon, Oxon, New York, NY, pp. 125–142.

Anthony, L. (2020) AntConc. Version 3.5.9. Tokyo, Japan, Waseda University. Available at: https://www.laurenceanthony.net/software/antconc/.

Anthony, L. (2023) Common statistics used in corpus linguistics. Available at: https://www.laurenceanthony.net/resources/statistics/common_statistics_used_in_corpus_linguistics.pdf. Accessed 10/1/2024.

Anyanwu, E. C. & Abana, I. (2020) A Speech Act Analysis of Public Speeches of Three African Presidents Amid Covid-19. *British Journal of English Language Linguistics* **8** (3), 10–18.

Apuge, M. & Warda, F. (2021) The Speech Acts of Requests in Cameroon Francophone English. *International Journal of English Language and Linguistics Research* **9** (4), 27–37.

Arsani, L., Juniartha, I. & Deni Ariyaningsih, N. (2021) An Analysis of Representative Speech Acts Used in Covid-19 Speech in Queen Elizabeth II. *Elysian Journal: English Literature, Linguistics and Translation Studies* **1** (1), 1–10.

Arsith, M. (2015) Political Discourse and the Theory of Speech Acts. *EIRP Proceedings* 10. Available at: https://proceedings.univ-danubius.ro/index.php/eirp/article/view/1653/1635. Accessed 6/10/2022.

Aryanto, B. (2020) Characteristics of Directive Speech Acts in the Dissemination of COVID-19 Mitigation Information in Japan. *Japanese Research on Linguistics, Literature and Culture* **3** (1), 13–26.

Aspinall, E. (2021) COVID-19 Timeline. British Foreign Policy Group (BFPG). Available at: https://bfpg.co.uk/2020/04/covid-19-timeline/. Accessed 1/18/2025.

Astira, M. (2023) Examining the Securitization of Muslim Immigrants in France Under the Anti- Separatist Act of President Emmanuel Macron. *Journal of Law and Social Transformation* **1** (1), 72–80.

Attamimy, H., Junining, E. & Khasanah, I. (2020) Speech Act Analysis of Jacinda Ardern about Covid-19. *Elite* **7** (2), 209–224.

Attia, S. (2022) Libya, the media and the language of violence: A Corpus-Assisted Discourse Analysis. *Research in Corpus Linguistics* **10** (1), 84–116.

Atuk, T. & Cannon, F. (2024) 'Monkeypox, where is your rage?': The racialization, sexualization, and securitization of global health. *Journal of Critical Public Health* **1** (2), 43–50.

Austin, J. L. (1962) *How to do Things With Words: The Williams James Lectures delivered at Harvard University in 1955*. Oxford University Press, Oxford.

Austin, J. R. (2023) "Some of you may die, but it's a sacrifice I am willing to make": Memes and the Social Media Critique by the UK Public in Response to COVID-19. In: Vakoch, D.A., Pollock, J.C., Caleb, A.M. (ed.) *COVID Communication*. Springer, Cham, pp. 233–241.

Ayoob, M. (1997) Defining Security: A Subaltern Realist Perspective. In: Krause, K. (ed.) *Critical Security Studies: Concepts and Strategies*. Hoboken, Routledge, pp. 260–286.

Badarneh, M. & Damiri, M. (2024) Criticizing for the public interest and aligning with others: How Jordanians constructed their online criticisms of lockdown breaches during the COVID-19 pandemic. *Pragmatics and Society* **15** (4), 557–583.

Baekkeskov, E., Rubin, O. & Öberg, P. (2021) Monotonous or pluralistic public discourse? Reason-giving and dissent in Denmark's and Sweden's early 2020 COVID-19 responses. *Journal of European Public Policy* **28** (8), 1321–1343.

Baele, S. J. & Jalea, D. (2023) Twenty five Years of Securitization Theory: A Corpus-based Review. *Political Studies Review* **21** (2), 376–389.

Baele, S. J. & Rousseau, E. (2023) At war or saving lives? On the securitizing semantic repertoires of Covid-19. *International Relations* **37** (2), 201–227.

Baker, P. (2009) The BE06 Corpus of British English and recent language change. *International Journal of Corpus Linguistics* **14** (3), 312–337.

Baker, P. (2020) Corpus-Assisted Discourse Analysis. In: Hart, C. (ed.) *Researching Discourse: A student guide*. Routledge, London and New York, pp. 124–142.

Baker, P., Gabrielatos, C., Khosravinik, M., Krzyżanowski, M., McEnery, T. & Wodak, R. (2008) A useful methodological synergy? Combining critical discourse analysis and corpus linguistics to examine discourses of refugees and asylum seekers in the UK press. *Discourse & Society* **19** (3), 273–306.

Balzacq, T. & Guzzini, S. (2015) Introduction: What kind of theory – if any – is securitization? *International Relations* **29** (1), 97–102.

Balzacq, T. (2005) The Three Faces of Securitization: Political Agency, Audience and Context. *European Journal of International Relations* **11** (2), 171–201.

Balzacq, T. (2011) A theory of securitization: Origins, core assumptions, and variants. In: Balzacq, T. (ed.) *Securitization theory: How security problems emerge and dissolve*. Routledge, Milton Park, Abingdon, Oxon, New York, pp. 1–30.

Balzacq, T. (2015) The 'Essence' of securitization: Theory, ideal type, and a sociological science of security. *International Relations* **29** (1), 103–113.

Balzacq, T. (2019) Securitization Theory: Past, Present, and Future. *Polity* **51** (2), 331–348.

Barahmeh, Y. & Fras, J. (2023) 'Every one of you is now a soldier': War metaphors in Jordanian official discourse during the COVID-19 pandemic. *Contemporary Levant* **8** (1), 87–99.

Baranova, L. L. (2021) English in the Pandemic: Changes and Challenges. *Professional Discourse & Communication* **3** (4), 84–90.

Baron, A., Rayson, P. & Archer, D. (2009) Word frequency and key word statistics in historical linguistics. *International Journal of English Studies* **20**, 41–67.

Barron, A. (2017) The speech act of 'offers' in Irish English. *World Englishes* **36** (2), 224–238.

Basra, S. & Thoyyibah, L. (2017) A Speech Act Analysis of Teacher Talk in an EFL Classroom. *International Journal of Education* **10** (1), 73–81.

Bayrak, F., Aktar, B., Aydas, B., Yilmaz, O., Alper, S. & Isler, O. (2024) Effective health communication depends on the interaction of message source and content: two experiments on adherence to COVID-19 measures in Türkiye. *Psychology & Health* **39** (13), 1847–1876.

Baysa-Barredo, J. M. (2020) Problematizing the Securitization of Covid-19 in Southeast Asia: A Necessary Step Towards an Inclusive, Rights-Centred Normal. Available at: https://shapesea.com/op-ed/problematizing-the-securitization-of-covid-19-in-southeast-asia-a-necessary-step-towards-an-inclusive-rights-centred-normal/. Accessed 12/29/2024.

Belkina, O. (2021) The Language of the Pandemic (Based on the French Language Materials). *SSRN Electronic Journal*.

Benoit, W. L. (1997) Image repair discourse and crisis communication. *Public Relations Review* **23** (2), 177–186.

Bilgin, P. (2011) The politics of studying securitization? The Copenhagen School in Turkey. *Security Dialogue* **42** (4–5), 399–412.

Binding, L. & McGuinness, A. (2020) Boris Johnson says...... *Sky News*, 26 January. https://news.sky.com/story/boris-johnson-says-britain-will-become-global-trail-blazing-country-after-brexit-11918062. Accessed 03/03/2026.

Biswas, S. (2012) Post-colonial security studies. In: Shepherd, L. J. (ed.) *Critical Approaches to Security: An Introduction to Theories and Methods*. Taylor and Francis, Hoboken, pp. 89–99.

BNC. British National Corpus. Available at: http://www.natcorp.ox.ac.uk/. Accessed 09/09/2024.

Bol, D. (2020) Nicola Sturgeon's daily Covid-19 media briefings cut to three days a week. *The Herald*, July 17. Available at: https://www.heraldscotland.com/news/18589505.nicola-sturgeons-daily-covid-19-media-briefings-cut-three-days-week. Accessed 6/13/2023.

Bourdieu, P. (1991) *Language and Symbolic Power*. Harvard University Press, Cambridge, MA.

Brown, P. & Levinson, S. C. (1987 [2016]) *Politeness: Some universals in language usage*, 25th printing 2016. Cambridge University Press, Cambridge.

Bühler, K. (1933) *Axiomatik der Sprachwissenschaften*. Klostermann, Frankfurt am Main.

Bülow, L., Diehr, A., Pfurtscheller, D. & Thome, S. (eds.) (2021) *Corona-Diskurse in und über Österreich*. Wiener Linguistische Gazette 90/91, Wien.

Burki, T. (2018) From health service to national identity: The NHS at 70. *The Lancet* **392** (10141), 15–17.

Burns, P. J. (2018) Constructing Stoplists for Historical Languages. *Digital Classics Online* **4** (2), 4–20.

Butler, J. (1996) Performativity's Social Magic. In: Schatzki, T. R. & Natter, W. (eds.) *The social and political body*. Guilford Press, New York, pp. 29–48.

Butler, J. (2021 [1997]) *Excitable speech: A politics of the performative*. Routledge Classics, London, New York.

Butler, M. & Wolf, Z. (2020) Introduction: Revisiting securitization and the 'constructivist turn' in security studies. In: Butler, M. J. (ed.) *Securitization Revisited. Contemporary Applications and Insights*. Routledge, Milton, pp. 1–25.

Buzan, B., Wæver, O. & Wilde, J. de (1998) *Security: A new Framework for Analysis*. London, Lynne Riener.

Cabinet Office (2023) COVID-19 – General public opinion tracker: Research and analysis. Government of the United Kingdom. Available at: https://www.gov.uk/government/publications/covid-19-general-public-opinion-tracker. Accessed 1/5/2025.

Callegari, E. (2023) Linguistic strategies to present complexity in a time of crisis. In: Thielemann, N. & Weiss, D. (eds.) *Remedies against the pandemic: How politicians communicate crisis management*. Amsterdam, John Benjamin, pp. 75–101.

Cambridge Dictionary (2024a) Press Release. Available at: https://dictionary.cambridge.org/dictionary/english/press-release. Accessed 11/6/2024.

Cambridge Dictionary (2024b) Prototypical. Available at: https://dictionary.cambridge.org/dictionary/english/prototypical. Accessed 20/08/2024.

Campbell, D. & Marsh, S. (2020) NHS could face 'horrendous choices' over who gets coronavirus care. *The Guardian,* December 30. Available at: https://www.theguardian.com/world/2020/dec/29/nhs-could-face-horrendous-choices-over-who-gets-coronavirus-care. Accessed 3/3/2025.

Canbazoğlu, A. (2020) The Effects of Public Service Announcements and Advertisements which Aired in the First Days of Covid-19 Coronovirüs Pandemic. *Turkish Studies (Journal of Turkish Studies)* **15** (6), 351–389.

Catalano, T. & Waugh, L. (2020) The Main Approaches to CDA/CDS. In: Catalano, T. & Waugh, L. R. (eds.) *Critical Discourse Analysis, Critical Discourse Studies and Beyond*. Springer International, Cham, pp. 155–217.

Chamberlain, E. F. (2023) COVID-19 as Metaphor: Fighting the Virus of Racism, Becoming the Vaccine. In: Vakoch, D. A., Pollock, J. C. & Caleb, A. M. (eds.) *COVID Communication*. Springer International, Cham, pp. 41–60.

Chang, C.-C., Yen, W.-T. & Liu, L.-Y. (2023) Fighting the Pandemic with "Shields": Successful COVID-19 Securitization and Mask Policy in Taiwan. *Journal of Asian and African Studie* **58** (2), 214–231.

Charrett, C. (2009) A Critical Application of Securitization Theory: Overcoming the Normative Dilemma of Writing Security. *SSRN Electronic Journal* (Working Paper No. 2009/7).

Charteris-Black, J. (2019) The Metaphors of Boris Johnson. In: Charteris-Black, J. (ed.). *Metaphors of Brexit*. Cham, Springer International, pp. 161–196.

Charteris-Black, J. (2021) *Metaphors of Coronavirus*. Cham, Springer International.

Cheng, W. (2012) *Exploring corpus linguistics. Language in action*. London, Routledge.

Christou, O. & Adamides, C. (2013) Energy securitization and desecuritization in the New Middle East. *Security Dialogue* **44** (5–6), 507–522.

Clarke, M. (2021) The trial of Dominic Cummings: Rules and reason in the pandemic. *Anthropology Today* **37** (2), 6–9.

Colomé-Menéndez, D., Koops, J. A. & Weggemans, D. (2021) A country of immigrants no more? The securitization of immigration in the National Security Strategies of the United States of America. *Global Affairs* **7** (1), 1–26.

Conrad, S. (2002) Corpus Linguistic Approaches for Discourse Analysis. *Annual Review of Applied Linguistics* **22**, 75–95.

Corbett, J. (2021) 'A Mild Dose of the Flu': The Discourse of the COVID-19 Crisis in Brazil and the Impact of the Pandemic on the Internationalization of Brazilian Higher Education. In: Zhao, S. X., Wong, J. H., Lowe, C., Monaco, E. & Corbett, J. (eds.) *COVID-19 Pandemic, Crisis Responses and the Changing World: Perspectives in Humanities and Social Sciences*. Singapore, Springer Singapore, pp. 207–225.

Côté, A. (2016) Agents without agency: Assessing the role of the audience in securitization theory. *Security Dialogue* **47** (6), 541–558.

Craig, D. (2020) Pandemic and its metaphors: Sontag revisited in the COVID-19 era. *European Journal of Cultural Studies* **23** (6), 1025–1032.

Cunningham, J. M. (2018) What's the Difference Between Great Britain and the United Kingdom? Available at: https://www.britannica.com/story/whats-the-difference-between-great-britain-and-the-united-kingdom. Accessed 10/26/2024.

Czerwionka, L., Dickerson, S. & Aragon-Bautista, R. (2021) Multimodal and Co-Constructed Speech Acts: Gratitude and Other Responses to Compliments and Gifts in Peninsular Spanish. In: Czerwionka, L., Showstack, R. & Liskin-Gasparro, J. E. (eds.) *Contexts of co-constructed discourse: Interaction, pragmatics, and second language applications*. Routledge, London, pp. 93–114.

Dau, D. & Ellis, K. (2023) From Bondi to Fairfield: NSW COVID-19 press conferences, health messaging, and social inequality. *Media International Australia* **188** (1), 34–51.

Davies, B., Lalot, F. & Peitz, L. et al. (2021) Changes in political trust in Britain during the COVID-19 pandemic in 2020: Integrated public opinion evidence and implications. Humanities and Social Sciences Communications **8** (1).

Davies, M. (2015) The Wikipedia Corpus. Available at: https://www.english-corpora.org/wiki/.

Davies, M. (2019) The Coronavirus Corpus. Available at: https://www.english-corpora.org/corona/.

Davies, M. (2021) Language and Covid-19. *International Journal of Corpus Linguistics* **26** (4), 583–598.

Davies, M. (2022) The Corpus of Contemporary American English (COCA). English-corpora.org. Available at: https://www.english-corpora.org/coca/.

Dayter, D. (2018) Self-praise online and offline. *Internet Pragmatics* **1** (1), 184–203.

Del Sarto, R. A. (2021) Sectarian securitization in the Middle East and the case of Israel. *International Affairs* **97** (3), 759–778.

Demirkol, A. (2022) An Empirical Analysis of Securitization Discourse in the European Union. *Migration Letters* **19** (3), 273–286.

Depala, R. (2023) Type Token Ratio in NLP. Available at: https://medium.com/@rajeswaridepala/empirical-laws-ttr-cc9f826d304d. Accessed 10/1/2024.

Derrida, J. (1972) Signature Event Context. *Margins of Philosophy*, 307–330.

Dickson, K., Aboltins, C., Pelly, J. & Jessup, R. L. (2023) Effective communication of COVID-19 vaccine information to recently-arrived culturally and linguistically diverse communities from the perspective of community engagement and partnership organisations: a qualitative study. *BMC health services research* **23** (1), 877.

Diehr, A. & Stiglbauer, R. (2021) (In-)Transparenz in der politischen Kommunikation der österreichischen Bundesregierung in ausgewählten Pressekonferenzen zur Corona-Ampel. In: Bülow, L., Diehr, A., Pfurtscheller, D. & Thome, S. (eds.) *Corona-Diskurse in und über Österreich*, pp. 39–74.

Dimari, G. & Papadakis, N. (2023) The securitization of the Covid-19 pandemic in Greece: a just or unjust securitization? *Quality & quantity* **57** (Suppl 1), 77–97.

Distler, W. (2021) The Governing of (In)Security. Politics and Securitisation in the Asian Context. International Quarterly for Asian Studies **52** (1–2), 5–13.

Doyle, D. (2023) Stopword Lists. *Ranks NL*. Available at: https://www.ranks.nl/stopwords. Accessed 11/16/2024.

Duarte, D. E. & Valença, M. M. (2021) Securitising Covid-19? The Politics of Global Health and the Limits of the Copenhagen School. *Contexto Internacional* **43** (2), 235–257.

Dubé, È., Labbé, F., Malo, B. & Pelletier, C. (2022) Public health communication during the COVID-19 pandemic: perspectives of communication specialists, healthcare professionals, and community members in Quebec, Canada. *Canadian journal of public health – Revue canadienne de sante publique* **113** (Suppl 1), 24–33.

Dylgjeri, A. (2017) Analysis of Speech Acts in Political Speeches. *European Journal of Social Sciences Studies* **3** (2), 19–26.

Ekpo, C. & Agorye, C. (2019) The Indigenous People of Biafra (IPOB) and the Setting of the "Jubril Al-Sudani" Agenda: A Qualitative Review of a Failed Securitization Move. *International Journal of Quantitative and Qualitative Research Methods* **7** (2), 1–17.

Ekron, Z. (2011) A critical and functional analysis of the mirror metaphor with reference to the media's responsibility towards society. *Global Media Journal African Edition* **2** (1), 80–87.

Engelkamp, S., Roepstorff, K. & Spencer, A. (2020) Visualizing Peace: The State of the Art. *Peace & Change* **45** (1), 5–27.

Farabi, N. & Saraswati, D. (2024) Securitization of Australian Migration during the Prime Minister Malcolm Turnbull's Presidency. *Journal of International Studies on Energy Affairs* **5** (2), 124–139.

Farnia, M. & Sattar, H. (2015) A Sociopragmatic Analysis of the Speech Act of Criticism by Persian Native Speakers. *International Journal of Humanities and Cultural Studies* **2** (3), 305–327.

Faturrochman, R. G., Darmawan, A. A. & Hadi, F. (2021) Teacher Talk in Scientific Approach in EFL Classroom: A Speech Acts Perspective. *SAGA: Journal of English Language Teaching and Applied Linguistics* **2** (1), 35–46.

Fazira, T. & Amri, Y. K. (2023) Analysis of Perlocutional Speech Acts on Whatsapp Chat. *LingLit Journal Scientific Journal for Linguistics and Literature* **4** (1), 32–39.

Fernández, Ó. (2024) The European Union's securitisation of global health: was COVID-19 a Zeitenwende? *European Security* **33** (3), 449–473.

Fernández-Pedemonte, D., Casillo, F. & Jorge-Artigau, A. I. (2020) Communi cating COVID-19: Metaphors We "Survive" By. *Tripodos* **2** (47), 145–159.

Filardo-Llamas, L. (2021) De tsunamis, olas, quijotes y KO-vid: Las metáforas de la pandemia a través de las viñetas. *Metode Science Studies Journal*, 14–20.

Finke, L. & Shichtman, M. (2007) Out of Mind, Out of Sight. *Arthuriana* **17** (1), 101–108.

Flowerdew, L. (2012) How is Corpus Linguistics Related to Discourse Analysis? *Corpora and Language Education* (Research and Practice in Applied Linguistics), 81–110.

Frame, A., Brachotte, G. & Selmi, A. (2022) A vos seringues: French Governmental Communication on COVID-19 Vaccination via Twitter. In: Maarek, P. J. (ed.) *Manufacturing Government Communication on Covid-19*. Springer International, Cham, pp. 371–395.

Frege, G. (1984) *Collected Papers on Mathematics, Logic, and Philosophy.* Edited by Brian McGuinness. Oxford: Blackwell.

Fridolfsson, C. & Elander, I. (2021) Between Securitization and Counter-Securitization: Church of Sweden Opposing the Turn of Swedish Government Migration Policy. *Politics, Religion & Ideology* **22** (1), 40–63.

Fuchs, J. (2021) Corona -Komposita und ‚Corona'-Konzepte in der Medienberichterstattung in Standardsprache und in Leichter Sprache. *Zeitschrift für germanistische Linguistik* **49** (2), 335–368.

Furkatovna, S., Jurabekovna, T. & Mamurjonovna, T. (2021) Gender aspects of politeness strategy in speech acts. *Linguistics and Culture Review* **5** (S2), 1488–1496.

Futák-Campbell, B. (2022) Facilitating crisis: Hungarian and Slovak securitization of migrants and their implications for EU politics. *International Politics* **59** (3), 541–561.

Garcia Guimarães, R. (2022) The securitization of health: on the protests against the Chinese "zero-COVID" strategy. UNIO – The Official Blog. Available at: https://officialblogofunio.com/2022/12/12/the-securitization-of-health-on-the-protests-against-the-chinese-zero-covid-strategy/. Accessed 3/8/2025.

Gayle, D. (2020) Thousands march in London in fourth anti-lockdown protest. *The Guardian,* October 24. Available at: https://www.theguardian.com/world/2020/oct/24/london-braces-for-fourth-protest-against-covid-19-restrictions. Accessed 1/20/2025.

Giritli Nygren, K. & Olofsson, A. (2021) Swedish exceptionalism, herd immunity and the welfare state: A media analysis of struggles over the nature and legitimacy of the COVID-19 pandemic strategy in Sweden. *Current Sociology* **69** (4), 529–546.

Gironzetti, E. (2021) Multimodal Resources in the Co-Construction of Humorous Discourse. In: Czerwionka, L., Showstack, R. & Liskin-Gasparro, J. E. (eds.) *Contexts of co-constructed discourse: Interaction, pragmatics, and second language applications*. Routledge, London, pp. 115–135.

Glomseth, R. & Boe, O. (2024) Norwegian Police Crisis Communication During the COVID-19 Pandemic. Digital Opportunities and Challenges. In: Ndlela, M. N. (ed.) *Organizational Communication in the Digital Era*. Springer Nature Switzerland, Cham, pp. 273–302.

Government of the United Kingdom (2024) News and communications. Available at: https://www.gov.uk/search/news-and-communications. Accessed 10/1/2024.

Gregory, A. & Campbell, D. (2022) Guardian's '33 hours' shows reality of NHS on edge of collapse, say doctors. *The Guardian,* December 14. Available at: https://www.theguardian.com/society/2022/dec/14/guardians-33-hours-shows-reality-of-nhs-on-edge-of-collapse-say-doctors. Accessed 3/30/2025.

Grice, H. P. (1975) Logic and Conversation. In: Cole, P. & Morgan, J. L. (eds.) *Syntax and Semantics*. New York, NY, Academic Press, pp. 41–58.

Griebel, T. & Vollmann, E. (2019) We can('t) do this: A corpus-assisted critical discourse analysis of migration in Germany. *Journal of Language and Politics* **18** (5), 671–697.

Griffiths, K. (2024) COVID-19 and Aboriginal and Torres Strait Islander People in Australia: Can Rhetoric Equal Action? In: Lewis, M., Govender, E. & Holland, K. (eds.) *Communicating COVID-19*. Springer International, Cham, pp. 189–202.

Guéraiche, W. (2022) The securitization of the COVID-19 crisis in the UAE. In: Guéraiche, W. & Alexander, K. (eds.) *Facets of security in the United Arab Emirates*. Routledge Taylor & Francis Group, London, New York, NY, pp. 271–285.

Günthner, S. (2021) WIR im interaktionalen Gebrauch: Zur Verwendung des Pronomens der 1. Person Plural in der institutionellen Kommunikation – am Beispiel onkologischer Aufklärungsgespräche. *Zeitschrift für germanistische Linguistik* **49** (2), 292–334.

Habermas, J. (1990) *Moral consciousness and communicative action*. Trans. Christian Lenhart and Sherry Weber Nicholson. Maldon, MA, Polity.

Hafner, C. A. & Sun, T. (2021) The 'team of 5 million': The joint construction of leadership discourse during the Covid-19 pandemic in New Zealand. *Discourse, Context & Media* **43**, 100523.

Hågemark, H. & Gärdenfors, P. (2025) Expressives, directives and assertions. Cognitive dimensions of speech acts. *Language & Communication* **101**, 84–104.

Hamed Ibrahim, N. M. (2022) The determinants of Jordan's stability case study: The arab spring (2011–2019) and the COVID-19 pandemic. *Asian Journal of Comparative Politics* **7** (3), 634–640.

Hanks, P. (2018) Types of Speech Acts. In: Fogal, D., Harris, D. & Moss, M. (eds.) *New work on speech acts*. Oxford, New York, Oxford University Press, pp. 123–143.

Hansen, L. (2020) Are 'core' feminist critiques of securitization theory racist? A reply to Alison Howell and Melanie Richter-Montpetit. *Security Dialogue* **51** (4), 378–385.

Hapal, K. (2021) The Philippines' COVID-19 Response. *Journal of Current Southeast Asian Affairs* **40** (2), 224–244.

Hardt, J. N., Harrington, C., Lucke, F. von, Estève, A. & Simpson, N. P. (eds.) (2023) *Climate Security in the Anthropocene: Exploring the Approaches of*

United Nations Security Council Member-States, 1st ed. 2023. Imprint Springer, Cham.

Hardt-Mautner, G. (1995) Only Connect. Critical Discourse Analysis and Corpus Linguistics. *UCREL Technical Paper* 6, 1–31. Available at: http://ucrel.lancs.ac.uk/papers/techpaper/vol6.pdf. Accessed 1/26/2021.

Harris, D., Fogal, D., Moss, M. (2018) Speech Acts: The Contemporary Theoretical Landscape. In: Daniel Fogal, Daniel W. Harris und Matt Moss (Hg.): New work on speech acts. Oxford, New York: Oxford University Press, pp. 1–39.

Hassan, H. A. (2022) The securitisation of COVID-19 in Africa: Socio-economic and political implications. *African Security Review* **31** (1), 19–32.

Hayek, L. (2024) Media Framing of Government Crisis Communication During Covid-19. *Media and Communication* **12**.

Hayes, J. (2011) Britain at War. Securitization, Identity, and the War in Iraq. *APSA 2011 Annual Meeting Paper*. Available at: https://papers.ssrn.com/sol3/papers.cfm?abstract_id=1900607. Accessed 12/12/2024.

Heaney, D. & Riboni, G. (2023) When a Liberal Use of Metaphor Is Really a Conservative One: The Case of Boris Johnson's Televised Press Releases. *Altre Modernità* (29), 173–194.

Heffner, G. (2020) Coronavirus: Sir Keir Starmer blames government 'failure' for new COVID-19 measures. *Sky News*, September 23. Available at: https://news.sky.com/story/coronavirus-keir-starmer-condemns-boris-johnsons-serial-incompetence-and-calls-for-fresh-economic-support-12079669. Accessed 1/20/2025.

Heidi, J. & Setyaningsih, N. (2024) Speech Act in a Courtroom: An Analysis of Chris Watts' Trial. *Allure Journal* **4** (1), 55–71.

Herrero-Arias, R., Halbostad, I. V. & Diaz, E. (2024) Norwegian "dugnad" as a rhetorical device in public health communication during the COVID-19 pandemic. A qualitative study from immigrant's perspectives. *Archives of public health = Archives belges de sante publique* **82** (1), 11.

Hoechner, H. & Salisu, I. (2022) Scapegoating the Usual Suspects? Pandemic Control and the Securitization of Qur'anic Education in Northern Nigeria. *Journal on Education in Emergencies* **8** (3), 108–135.

Hoffman, A. (2020) The Securitization of the Coronavirus Crisis in the Middle East. In: *The COVID-19 Pandemic in the Middle East and North Africa*. POMEPS Studes 39, pp. 10–14.

Holtgraves, T. (2021) Understanding Miscommunication: Speech Act Recognition in Digital Contexts. *Cognitive science* **45** (10), e13023.

Holtgraves, T. (2024) Emoji, Speech Acts, and Perceived Communicative Success. *Journal of Language and Social Psychology* **43** (1), 83–103.

Holze, R. (2023) Shambolic blunder: Boris Johnson's communication of failure during the Covid-19 pandemic. In: Thielemann, N. & Weiss, D. (eds.) *Remedies against the pandemic: How politicians communicate crisis management*. Amsterdam, John Benjamin, pp. 171–197.

Holze, R. (2026) Johnson Pandemic Corpus 2020 (JPanC20) [Data set]. ZENODO. https://doi.org/10.5281/zenodo.15591245.

Hong, S.-A. (2023) COVID-19 vaccine communication and advocacy strategy: A social marketing campaign for increasing COVID-19 vaccine uptake in South Korea. *Humanities and Social Sciences Communications* **10** (1), 109.

Horton, R. (2023) Offline: Boris Johnson and COVID-19—more light than heat. The Lancet **402**, 2277.

Howell, A. & Richter-Montpetit, M. (2020) Is securitization theory racist? Civilizationism, methodological whiteness, and antiblack thought in the Copenhagen School. *Security Dialogue* **51** (1), 3–22.

Huang, L. (2021) Developing a multimodal corpus of speech acts in situated discourse. In: Huang, L. (ed.) *Toward multimodal pragmatics: A study of illocutionary force in Chinese situated discourse*. Routledge, London, New York, pp. 109–159.

Hussein, A. & Noori, B. (2023) Speech Acts Used in Covid-19 English and Arabic News Reports. *Al-Adab Journal* **145** (1), 1–14.

Huysmans, J. (2011) What's an Act? On Security Speech Acts and Little Security Nothings. *Security Dialogue* **42**, 371–381.

Hvitfeldt, E. & Silge, J. (2021) *Supervised Machine Learning for Text Analysis in R*. Chapman and Hall/CRC, Boca Raton.

Imran, M. A. & Ahmed, Z. (2025) 'We're in this together' – COVID-19 statements by Boris Johnson. A discourse analysis. *Media International Australia* **197** (1), 242–258.

Innes, A. (2024) Un-siloing securitization: An intersectional intervention. *International Politics*, 1–22.

Institute for Government (2022) Timeline of UK government coronavirus lockdowns and restrictions. Available at: https://www.instituteforgovernment.org.uk/data-visualisation/timeline-coronavirus-lockdowns. Accessed 1/18/2025.

Ivić, S. & Petrović, R. (2020) The Rhetoric of Othering in a Time of Pandemic. Labeling COVID-19 as a "Foreign Virus" in Public Discourse. *Kultura Polisa* **17** (43), 421–433.

Jäger, S. (2024) Abgehängt von Chinas Elektroautos: VW, BMW und Mercedes steuern auf eine Katastrophe in China zu. *Finanzmarktwelt*. Available at: https://finanzmarktwelt.de/vw-bmw-und-mercedes-steuern-auf-eine-katastrophe-in-china-zu-326176/. Accessed 12/28/2024.

Jarren, O. & Donges, P. (2011) *Politische Kommunikation in der Mediengesellschaft: Eine Einführung*, 3rd edition. Wiesbaden, VS Verl. für Sozialwiss.

Jaworska, S. & Vásquez, C. (2022) COVID-19 and the discursive practices of political leadership: Introduction. *Discourse, Context & Media* **47**, 100605.

Jaworska, S. (2016) A comparative corpus-assisted discourse study of the representations of hosts in promotional tourism discourse. *Corpora* **11** (1), 83–111.

Jaworska, S. (2021) Competence and collectivity: The discourse of Angela Merkel's media communications during the first wave of the pandemic. *Discourse, Context & Media* **42**, 1–9.

Jegede, O. O. (2025) Speech Acts in the Digital Sphere: A Corpus-Based Exploration of Interactional Dynamics on Social Media Platforms. *Corpus-based Studies across Humanities* **2** (2), 359–383.

Johnson, B. & Leyen, U. von der (2020) *Joint Statement from UK Prime Minister Boris Johnson and European Commission President von der Leyen: 7 December 2020*.

Johnson, B. (2020au) *The Future Relationship between the UK and the EU: Written statement to Parliament*. 3 February 2020, London.

Johnson, Boris [@BorisJohnson], (2020, 27 March) Over the last 24 hours I have developed mild symptoms and tested positive for coronavirus. I am now self-isolating [Tweet]. *X (Twitter)*. https://x.com/BorisJohnson/status/1243496858095411200 [08.11.2024].

Jones, R. H. (2021) *Viral Discourse*. Cambridge, Cambridge University Press.

Jucker, A. H. (2024) *Speech acts: Discursive, multimodal, diachronic*. Cambridge University Press, Cambridge.

Just, M., Saraceno, J. & Crigler, A. (2022) Trump Confronts COVID in Press Briefings and on Twitter. In: Maarek, P. J. (ed.) *Manufacturing Government Communication on Covid-19*. Springer International, Cham, pp. 215–230.

Kádár, D. Z. & Zhang, S. (2019) (Im)politeness and alignment. *Acta Linguistica Academica* **66** (2), 229–249.

Kamil, M. b. A. & Bahrn, F. b. S. (2020) A Speech Act Analysis of the Prime Minister's Speech Pertaining to the Movement Control Order (MCO) to Address the Covid-19 Pandemic in Malaysia. *International Journal of Modern Languages and Applied Linguistics* **4** (4), 1–13.

Kartika, D., Rahardi, R. K., Aziz, M. & Rahmat, W. (2023) Depicting reflections of power on illocutionary acts of Japanese Prime Minister Shinzō Abe's speeches on Covid-19. *Indonesian Journal of Applied Linguistics* **13** (2), 283–292.

Kartoglu, U. & Pala, K. (2023) Evaluation of COVID-19 pandemic management in Türkiye. *Frontiers in Public Health* **11**, 1–12.

Kaunert, C. & Ezeokafor, E. (2022) Ontological Securitization of Health in Africa: The HIV/AIDS, Ebola and COVID-19 Pandemics and the Foreign Virus. *Social Sciences* **11** (8), 352.

Kembo, S. (2024) A Comparative Analysis of Government Social Media-Based Crisis and Risk Communication during the COVID-19 Health Crisis. In: Jakaza, E., Mangeya, H. & Mhute, I. (eds.) *The Palgrave Handbook of Language and Crisis Communication in Sub-Saharan Africa*. Springer International, Cham, pp. 343–365.

Khaya, Y. (2024) The Taxonomy of Denial as a Speech Act. *International Journal of Linguistics, Literature & Translation* **7** (3), 141–145.

Kikkawa, T. (2024) Jordan's Regime Security Under the COVID-19 Pandemic: Securitisation Against Visible and Invisible Threats. *Alternatives: Global, Local, Political*.

Kirby, J. (2023) The way Boris Johnson made decisions was 'unique' – Sir Chris Whitty. *Independent*, November 21. Available at: https://www.independent.co.uk/news/uk/boris-johnson-jonathan-vantam-chris-whitty-government-patrick-vallance-b2451093.html. Accessed 10/10/2024.

Kirk, J. & McDonald, M. (2021) The Politics of Exceptionalism: Securitization and COVID-19. *Global Studies Quarterly* **1** (3), 1–12.

Kirk, J. (2023) *More than a health crisis: Securitization and the US response to the 2013–2016 Ebola outbreak*. Cambridge, London, The MIT Press.

Kneuer, M. & Wallaschek, S. (2023) Framing COVID-19: Public Leadership and Crisis Communication By Chancellor Angela Merkel During the Pandemic in 2020. *German Politics* **32** (4), 686–709.

Knock, E. S., Whittles, L. K. & Lees, J. A. et al. (2021) Key epidemiological drivers and impact of interventions in the 2020 SARS-CoV-2 epidemic in England. *Science translational medicine* **13** (602), 1–11.

Kretchmar, R. S. (2001) A Functionalist Analysis of Game Acts: Revisiting Searle. *Journal of the Philosophy of Sport* **28** (2), 160–172.

Kupolati, O., Adebileje, A. & Adeleke, A. (2021) "Someone has been coronated" Nigerian English lexical innovations in the COVID-19 Pandemic. *Cogent Arts & Humanities* **8** (1), 1–13.

Kuteleva, A. & Clifford, S. J. (2021) Gendered securitisation: Trump's and Putin's discursive politics of the COVID-19 pandemic. *European Journal of International Security* **6** (3), 301–317.

Lamontagne, M. (2024) Securitization versus sovereignty? Multi-level governance, scientific objectivation, and the discourses of the Canadian and American heads of state during the first wave of the COVID-19 pandemic. *International journal (Toronto, Ont.)* **79** (3), 369–396.

Larsson, O. L. (2022) The Swedish Covid-19 strategy and voluntary compliance: Failed securitisation or constitutional security management? *European Journal of International Security* **7** (2), 226–247.

Laruelle, M., Alexseev, M. & Buckley, C. et al. (2021) Pandemic Politics in Eurasia: Roadmap for a New Research Subfield. *Problems of Post-Communism* **68** (1), 1–16.

Léonard, S. & Kaunert, C. (2020) *Refugees, security and the European Union*. London, New York Routledge Taylor & Francis Group.

Lewis, D. (1979) Scorekeeping in a language game. *Journal of Philosophical Logic* **8** (1), 339–359.

Lilleker, D. & Stoeckle, T. (2021) The challenges of providing certainty in the face of wicked problems: Analysing the UK government's handling of the COVID-19 pandemic. *Journal of public affairs* **21** (4), 1–10.

Lilleker, D., Coman, I., Gregor, M. & Novelli, E. (eds.) (2021) *Political communication and COVID-19: Governance and rhetoric in times of crisis*. Routledge Taylor & Francis Group, London, New York.

Lin, P. & Chen, Y. (2020) Multimodality I: speech, prosody and gestures. In: Adolphs, S. & Knight, D. (eds.) *The Routledge handbook of English language and digital humanities*. Routledge, Abingdon, Oxon, New York, NY, pp. 66–84.

Liu, B. F., Iles, I. A. & Herovic, E. (2020) Leadership under Fire: How Governments Manage Crisis Communication. *Communication Studies* **71** (1), 128–147.

Lowe, C. & Barber, B. (2021) The "Perfect Storm": A Failed Response to the Pandemic in the United States. In: Zhao, S. X., Wong, J. H., Lowe, C., Monaco, E. & Corbett, J. (eds.) *COVID-19 Pandemic, Crisis Responses and the Changing World: Perspectives in Humanities and Social Sciences*, 1st ed. 2021. Springer Singapore; Imprint Springer, Singapore, pp. 189–205.

Lowe, M., Harmon, S., Kholina, K., Parker, R. & Graham, J. E. (2022) Public health communication in Canada during the COVID-19 pandemic. *Canadian journal of public health – Revue canadienne de sante publique* **113** (Suppl 1), 34–45.

Lucini, B. (2025) Crisis Communication and Governance: Lessons Learned from Covid – 19 Pandemic in Italy. *Public Organization Review*, 1–16.

Lukacovic, M. (2022) The Normative Dimension of Securitization as a Strategic Crisis Communication Theory: Lessons from the COVID-19 Pandemic in Central & Eastern Europe. *Social Communications: Theory and PracticeS* **14** (1), 197–209.

Lukacovic, M. N. (2020) "Wars" on COVID-19 in Slovakia, Russia, and the United States: Securitized Framing and Reframing of Political and Media Communication Around the Pandemic. *Frontiers in Communication* **5**.

Ma'yuuf, H. H. & Ghitheeth, H. H. (2021) Directive and Assertive Speech Acts in Selected Covid 19 News. *Journal of Arts, Literature, Humanities and Social Sciences* **63**, 400–410.

Maher, J. (2024) *The World of Coronaspeak: Mockdown, PCR and Surgeon's Finger*. Cambridge, Cambridge Scholars Publishing.

Majeed, R. M. (2022) A Pragmatic Analysis of Illocutionary Act in a Selected Presidential Speech on COVID-19. *Journal of the College of languages* **0** (45), 84–107.

Malamatidou, S. (2020) Multimodality II: text and image. In: Adolphs, S. & Knight, D. (eds.) *The Routledge handbook of English language and digital humanities*. Routledge, Abingdon, Oxon, New York, NY, pp. 85–107.

Manzoor, A. (2017) Social Media as Mirror of Society. In: Trivedi, S. K., Dey, S., Kumar, A. & Panda, T. K. (eds.) *Handbook of research on advanced data mining techniques and applications for business intelligence*. Hershey, PA, USA, Business Science Reference, pp. 128–141.

Marchi, A. & Taylor, C. (2018) Introduction. In: Taylor, C. & Marchi, A. (eds.) *Corpus approaches to discourse: A critical review*. Abingdon, Routledge, pp. 1–15.

Marciano, A. & Yadlin, A. (2022) Media coverage of COVID-19 state surveillance in Israel: The securitization and militarization of a civil-medical crisis. *Media, Culture & Society* **44** (3), 445–463.

Marsen, S. & Ali-Chand, Z. (2022) 'We all have a role to play': A comparative analysis of political speech acts on the COVID19 crisis in the South Pacific. *Communication Research and Practice* **8** (1), 19–35.

Martini, A. & Russo, A. (2025) The pandemic sovereign: how the war against the virus redefined sovereignty in Italy and Spain. *Critical Military Studies*, 1–24.

Mason, R. (2020) UK could have Europe's worst coronavirus death rate, says adviser. *The Guardian*, April 12. https://www.theguardian.com/world/2020

/apr/12/uk-could-have-europes-worst-coronavirus-death-rate-says-pandemic-expert. Accessed 03/03/2026.

Matthews, A. (2021) Sociotechnical imaginaries in the present and future university: a corpus-assisted discourse analysis of UK higher education texts. *Learning, Media and Technology* **46** (2), 204–217.

Mautner, G. (2007) Mining large corpora for social information: The case of elderly. *Language in Society* **36** (01).

Mautner, G. (2016) Checks and Balances. How corpus linguistics can contribute to CDA. In: Wodak, R. & Meyer, M. (eds.) (2016) *Methods of Critical Discourse*. London, Sage, pp. 154–179.

Mbogoh, A. & Mwatela, R. (2020) Public Health or Security Issue: An Analysis of Kenya's Response to the COVID-19 Pandemic. In: Obika, J., Ndayisaba, L., Trouille, J.-M. & Trouille, H. (eds.) *Africa, the European Union and China Towards a New Global Order – From Pandemic to Renewed Integration and Global Cooperation?* Special Issue 2020 – Part 3, Chisinau, pp. 165–188.

McAllister, I. (2007) The Personalization of Politics. In: Dalton, E. & Klingemann, H.-D. (eds.). *Oxford handbook of political behavior.* Oxford/New York, Oxford University Press, pp. 571–588.

McClaughlin, E.; Nichele, E.; Adolphs, S.; Barnard, P.; Clos, J.; Knight, D.; McAuley, D. & Lang, Alexandra (2021) Public health messaging by political leaders: A corpus linguistic analysis of COVID-19 speeches delivered by Boris Johnson. Research Highlight Report July 2021. Available at: https://orca.cardiff.ac.uk/id/eprint/143719/1/coronavirus_discourses_SR02.pdf. Accessed 5/31/2023.

McDonald, M. (2008) Securitization and the Construction of Security. *European Journal of International Relations* **14** (4), 563–587.

McGuire, D., Cunningham, J. E. A., Reynolds, K. & Matthews-Smith, G. (2020) Beating the virus: an examination of the crisis communication approach taken by New Zealand Prime Minister Jacinda Ardern during the Covid-19 pandemic. *Human Resource Development International* **23** (4), 361–379.

McQuail, D. (2005) *McQuail's Mass Communication Theory*. Sage, London.

Medrado, A. & Cabral, A. (2022) Contrasting Federal and State Government Communication on Facebook in Brazil: Contradictory Messages and Realities. In: Maarek, P. J. (ed.) *Manufacturing Government Communication on Covid-19*. Springer International, Cham, pp. 175–198.

Meibauer, J. (2022) Pragmatik und Recht: Kriminelle Sprechakte. *Linguistische Treffen in Wrocław* **21** (1), 143–163.

Mendes, C., Santos, L. B. d. & Souza, M. de (2020) Climate change, vulnerability and securitization. *Revista Brasileira de Política Internacional* **63** (1), 1–26.

Mercer, D. (2020) COVID-19: More than 150 arrests as anti-lockdown protesters clash with police in London. *Sky News,* November 29. Available at: https://news.sky.com/story/covid-19-anti-lockdown-protesters-clash-with-police-in-london-12144977. Accessed 1/20/2025.

Messerli, T., Dayter, D., Leuckert, S., Liimatta, A., Mahler, H., Bohmann, A., Kozma, G. & Tosin, R. (2025) Digital debating cultures: communicative practices on Reddit. *Digital Scholarship in the Humanities* **fqaf005**.

Mohammed, M. J. (2023) A Speech Act Approach to Translation of English Politeness Formulas into Arabic. مجلة آداب الفراهيدي **15** (53), 589–602.

Mollin, S. (2007) The Hansard Hazard: Gauging the Accuracy of British Parliamentary Transcripts. *Corpora* **2** (2), 187–210.

Molnár, A., Takács, L. & Jakusné Harnos, É. (2020) Securitization of the COVID-19 pandemic by metaphoric discourse during the state of emergency in Hungary. *International Journal of Sociology and Social Policy* **40** (9/10), 1167–1182.

Monaco, E., Tang, K. C., Cheng, W., Liu, H. & Pan, B. (2021) Actions Across Government and COVID-19: The Experience of Mainland China, Macao and Hong Kong. In: Zhao, S. X., Wong, J. H., Lowe, C., Monaco, E. & Corbett, J. (eds.) *COVID-19 Pandemic, Crisis Responses and the Changing World: Perspectives in Humanities and Social Sciences*. Springer Singapore, Singapore, pp. 57–82.

Morales-Ramírez, I. & Perini, A. (2014) Discovering Speech Acts in Online Discussions: A Tool-supported method. In: Nurcan, S. & Pimenidis, E. (eds.) *Proceedings of the CAiSE'2014 Forum at the 26th International Conference on Advanced Information Systems Engineering (CAiSE)*, pp. 137–144.

Morgan, M. (2020). Why meaning-making matters: The case of the UK Government's COVID-19 response. *American Journal of Cultural Sociology* **8**, 270–323

Mukubano, J. (2020) Burundi et le COVID-19: Scenarii de Fragilité. In: Obika, J., Ndayisaba, L., Trouille, J.-M. & Trouille, H. (eds.) *Africa, the European Union and China Towards a New Global Order – From Pandemic to Renewed Integration and Global Cooperation?* Special Issue 2020 – Part 3, Chisinau, pp. 189–200.

Murray, J. (2020) Covid vaccine: UK woman becomes first in world to receive Pfizer jab. *The Guardian*, December 08. Available at: https://www.theguardian.com/world/2020/dec/08/coventry-woman-90-first-patient-to-receive-covid-vaccine-in-nhs-campaign. Accessed 11/4/2024.

Musolff, A. (2022) 'War against Covid-19'. Is the pandemic management as war metaphor helpful or hurtful? In: Musolff, A., Breeze, R., Kondo, K. et al.

(eds.). *Pandemic and crisis discourse.* Communicating COVID-19 and public health strategy. London, England: Bloomsbury, pp. 307–320.

Muttaqin, U., Yulianita, N. G. & Yulianti, U. H. (2020) Speech Acts and Its Translation Accuracy in Bilingual Fables. *J-Lalite: Journal of English Studies* **1** (2), 161–172.

Nartowski, R. O., Huby, L., Topham, R., Golen, S., Brückner, K., Hanigan, G., Saleem, H., Bielska, I. A., Shepherd, P. & Feltis, S. (2020) From 'herd immunity' to 'stay home' to 'stay alert': United Kingdom's response to COVID-19. *Zdrowie Publiczne i Zarządzanie* **18** (1), 46–58.

Nasrullah, R. & Gustini, D. R. (2022) Digital Speech Acts on Social Media: The Content Ethnographic of Audiences Response to the Publication of Illegal Online Loans on @Ojkindonesia's Instagram Account. *Jurnal Komunikasi Ikatan Sarjana Komunikasi Indonesia* **7** (2), 450–459.

Neo, R. (2020) Securitization of the President. Trump as a National Security Threat. *Cambridge Review of International Affairs*, 1–22.

Nervino, E., Lan, G. & Cheung, J. O. (2025) Sustainability as a business opportunity: A corpus-assisted discourse analysis of sustainable finance discourse. *Applied Linguistics Review.*

Newton, K. (2020) Government Communications, Political Trust and Compliant Social Behaviour: The Politics of Covid-19 in Britain. *The Political Quarterly* **91** (3), 502–513.

Njuki, E. & Ireri, H. K. (2021) Positive and Negative Politeness Strategies Used by Kenya's Members of National Assembly. *OALib* **08** (08), 1–20.

Nkang, O. N. & Bassey, O. B. (2022) Securitization of Global Health Pandemic and Reiterating the Relevance of 2005 International Health Regulations: COVID-19 and Human Security in Africa. *African Journal of Empirical Research* **3** (1), 36–48.

Nord, L. (2022) No Lockdown Please, We Are Swedish: How the Middle Way Country Became an Extreme Case of Government Communication. In: Maarek, P. J. (ed.) *Manufacturing Government Communication on Covid-19.* Springer International, Cham, pp. 107–121.

Nossek, H. (2022) Government Communication Policy for Dealing with the COVID-19, the Case of Israel: How to Explain to Groups with Unique Communication Characteristics a Universal Phenomenon. In: Maarek, P. J. (ed.) *Manufacturing Government Communication on Covid-19.* Springer International, Cham, pp. 199–211.

Nurkhamidah, N. (2020) Illocutionary speech acts on Donald Trump's speech in addressing the covid-19 breakout. *Journal of Research on English and Language Learning (J-REaLL)* **1** (2), 119.

Nyman, J. (2012) Securitization theory. In: Shepherd, L. J. (ed.) *Critical Approaches to Security: An Introduction to Theories and Methods*. Hoboken, Taylor and Francis, pp. 51–62.

O'Halloran, K., Tan, S. & K. L. E., M. (2014) Multimodal pragmatics. In: Schneider, K. P. & Barron, A. (eds.) *Pragmatics of Discourse*. De Gruyter Mouton, Boston, pp. 239–268.

Okoli, A. C. & Ngwu, E. C. (2022) Of Gainers, Losers, and Victims: COVID-19 and Securitized Lockdown in Nigeria in Early 2020. *PanAfrican Journal of Governance and Development* **3** (2), 62–84.

Olsson, E.-K. & Eriksson, M. (2020) Crisis communication in public organizations. In: Frandsen, F. & Johansen, W. (eds.) *Crisis Communication*. Berlin, de Gruyter, pp. 419–438.

Olsson, E.-K. (2014) Crisis Communication in Public Organisations: Dimensions of Crisis Communication Revisited. *Journal of Contingencies and Crisis Management* **22** (2), 113–125.

Olza, I., Koller, V., Ibarretxe-Antuñano, I., Pérez-Sobrino, P. & Semino, E. (2021) The #ReframeCovid initiative. *Metaphor and the Social World* **11** (1), 98–120.

Omelicheva, M. Y. & Markowitz, L. P. (2022) COVID-19 in Central Asia: (De-)Securitization of a Health Crisis? *Problems of Post-Communism* **69** (1), 92–102.

Önsoy, M. & Pelit, S. (2022) The Securitization and De-Securitization of the Name Issue Between Greece and North Macedonia: A North Macedonian Perspective. *Karadeniz Araştırmaları* **19** (74), 329–345.

Osah, G., Ojo, O., Eti, C. & Ali, A. (2020) Covid 19, Securitization and the Nigerian State: A political-economy perspective. *Global Journal of Applied, Management and Social Sciences* **20**, 120–130.

Oshitani, H. (2022) COVID lessons from Japan: the right messaging empowers citizens. *Nature* **605** (7911), 589.

Osler, L. & Zahavi, D. (2022) Sociality and Embodiment: Online Communication During and After Covid-19. *Foundations of science*, 1–18.

Østebø, M. T., Østebø, T. & Tronvoll, K. (2021) Health and politics in pandemic times: COVID-19 responses in Ethiopia. *Health policy and planning* **36** (10), 1681–1689.

Owusu, G. (2021) Fighting the Invisible Enemy—COVID-19: How Ghana Fared. In: Zhao, S. X., Wong, J. H., Lowe, C., Monaco, E. & Corbett, J. (eds.)

COVID-19 Pandemic, Crisis Responses and the Changing World: Perspectives in Humanities and Social Sciences. Springer Singapore, Singapore, pp. 173–187.

Ozoliņa, Ž. & Struberga, S. (2022) Crisis Communication During the Pandemic: Latvia's Case. In: Maarek, P. J. (ed.) *Manufacturing Government Communication on Covid-19*. Springer International, Cham, pp. 59–77.

Pablos-Ortega, C. de (2020) Directive Speech Acts in English and Spanish Filmspeak. *Pragmática Sociocultural / Sociocultural Pragmatics* **8** (1), 105–125.

Palosaari, T. & Tynkkynen, N. (2015) Arctic securitization and climate change. In: Hønneland, G. & Jensen, L. C. (eds.) *Handbook of the politics of the Arctic*. Edward Elgar, Cheltenham, pp. 87–104.

Pan, G. (2024) Politics of Decisionism: Carl Schmitt, Securitization and the Logic of China's COVID-19. *SSRN Electronic Journal*, 1–24.

Partington, A. (2006) Metaphors, Motifs and Similes across Discourse Types. In: A. Stefanowitsch & S. T. Gries (eds.) *Corpus-based approaches to metaphor and metonymy.: Trends in Linguistics*. Berlin, de Gruyter, pp. 267–304.

Partington, A., Duguid, A. & Taylor, C. (2013) *Patterns and meanings in discourse: Theory and practice in corpus-assisted discourse studies (CADS)*. John Benjamins, Amsterdam.

Paton, C. (2021) 'We did everything we could': An account of toxic leadership. *The International journal of health planning and management* **36** (6), 1972–1989.

Paton, C. (2022) World-beating? Testing Britain's Covid response and tracing the explanation. *Health economics, policy, and law* **17** (2), 238–245.

Patterson, T. (2008) The News as a Reflection of Public Opinion. In: Donsbach, W. (ed.) *The SAGE handbook of public opinion research*. Los Angeles, Sage, pp. 34–41.

Paun, A., Sargeant, J., Shuttleworth, K. & Nice, A. (2020) Coronavirus and devolution. *Institute for Government.* Available at: https://www.institutef orgovernment.org.uk/article/explainer/coronavirus-and-devolution. Accessed 10/26/2024.

Pearse, H. (2020). Deliberation, citizen science and covid-19. *The Political Quarterly* **91** (3), 571–577.

Pei, J. & Cheng, L. (2024) Representations of 5G in the Chinese and British press: A corpus-assisted critical discourse analysis. *Humanities and Social Sciences Communications* **11** (1), 1–12.

Peoples, C. & Vaughan-Williams, N. (2021) *Critical Security Studies: An introduction*, 3rd edition. London, New York, Routledge.

Perera, K. & Makoni, S. (2019) The Securitization of Language Education. *Applied Linguistics* **40** (5), 859–863.

Pérez-Sobrino, P., Semino, E., Ibarretxe-Antuñano, I., Koller, V. & Olza, I. (2022) Acting like a Hedgehog in Times of Pandemic Metaphorical Creativity in the #reframecovid Collection. *Metaphor and Symbol* **37** (2), 127–139.

Pfrimer, M. & Barbosa, R. (2020) Brazil's war on COVID-19: Crisis, not conflict—Doctors, not generals. *Dialogues in Human Geography* **10** (2), 137–140.

Picheta, R. (2020) Boris Johnson issues stay-at-home order, sending UK into lockdown to fight coronavirus pandemic. *CNN*, March 24. Available at: https://edition.cnn.com/2020/03/23/uk/uk-coronavirus-lockdown-gbr-intl/index.html. Accessed 09/09/2024.

Pojanapunya, P. & Watson Todd, R. (2018) Log-likelihood and odds ratio: Keyness statistics for different purposes of keyword analysis. *Corpus Linguistics and Linguistic Theory* **14** (1), 133–167.

Pollak, G., Decker, J.-O. & Dengel, A. et al. (2018) Interdisziplinäre Grundlagen der Information and Media Literacy (IML): Theoretische Begründung und (hochschul-)didaktische Realisierung – Ein Positionspapier. *PAradigma: Beiträge aus Forschung und Lehre aus dem Zentrum für Lehrerbildung und Fachdidaktik, Bd. 9 (2018)PAradigma: Beiträge aus Forschung und Lehre aus dem Zentrum für Lehrerbildung und Fachdidaktik* (9), 14–129.

Pour-Ahmadi, H. & Mohseni, S. (2012) The Obama Administration and Securitization of Iran's Nuclear Energy Program. *Iranian Review of Foreign Affairs* **3** (2), 143–174.

Prastio, B., Ibrahim, A. S., Susanto, G. & Nurzafira, I. (2021) Pattern of indirect directive speech acts on online advertisements. *Bahasa dan Seni: Jurnal Bahasa, Sastra, Seni, dan Pengajarannya* **49** (2).

Proudfoot, A. G., O'Brien, B., Schilling, R., Gould, D. W. & McGlennan, A. (2021) Rapid establishment of a COVID-19 critical care unit in a convention centre: The Nightingale Hospital London experience. *Intensive care medicine* **47** (3), 349–351.

Raheem, B. R. & Nehal, R. (2021) A Pragmatic Study of Speech Acts Pertaining to Health Advice in Covid-19 Pandemic. *Journal for the Study of English Linguistics* **9** (1), 103.

Rajagopalan, K. (2000) On Searle [on Austin] on language. *Language & Communication* **20** (4), 347–391.

Rajandran, K. (2020) 'A Long Battle Ahead': Malaysian and Singaporean Prime Ministers Employ War Metaphors for COVID-19. *Journal of Language Studies* **20** (3), 261–267.

Rana, M. S. & Riaz, A. (2023) Securitization of the Rohingya Refugees in Bangladesh. *Journal of Asian and African Studies* **58** (7), 1274–1290.

Rathnayake, C., Smith, A. & Higgins, M. (2023) Emergent Twitter publics through political scandal. *Journal of Language and Politics* **22** (4), 458–484.

Rauchfleisch, A., Vogler, D. & Eisenegger, M. (2021) Public Sphere in Crisis Mode: How the COVID-19 Pandemic Influenced Public Discourse and User Behaviour in the Swiss Twitter-sphere. *Javnost (Ljubljana, Slovenia)* **28** (2), 129–148.

Raupp, J. (2022) "The Situation Is Serious": Angela Merkel's Crisis Communication in the COVID-19 Pandemic. In: Maarek, P. J. (ed.) *Manufacturing Government Communication on Covid-19*. Springer International, Cham, pp. 231–251.

Rawlinson, K. (2020) 'This enemy can be deadly': Boris Johnson invokes wartime language. *The Guardian,* March 17. Available at: https://www.theguardian.com/world/2020/mar/17/enemy-deadly-boris-johnson-invokes-wartime-language-coronavirus. Accessed 7/12/2024.

Razak, F., Shin, S., Naylor, C. D. & Slutsky, A. S. (2022) Canada's response to the initial 2 years of the COVID-19 pandemic: a comparison with peer countries. *CMAJ Canadian Medical Association journal = journal de l'Association medicale canadienne* **194** (25), E870-E877.

Rebolledo, M. & Rodríguez-Virgili, J. (2022) National Leadership Versus Regional Command: The Case of the Spanish COVID-19 Crisis. In: Maarek, P. J. (ed.) *Manufacturing Government Communication on Covid-19*. Springer International, Cham, pp. 125–145.

Reuters (2020) UK's test and trace system not had wanted impact, PM Johnson says. *Reuters*, 6 November 2020. Available at: https://www.reuters.com/article/us-health-coronavirus-britain-johnson-te-idUSKBN27L2J9. Accessed 3/3/2026.

Ridanpää, J. (2014) 'Humour is Serious' as a Geopolitical Speech Act: IMDb Film Reviews of Sacha Baron Cohen's The Dictator. *Geopolitics* **19** (1), 140 – 160.

Roberts, L. (2022) UK to face 'prolonged period' of excess deaths following pandemic, say health chiefs. *The Telegraph,* December 01. Available at: https://www.telegraph.co.uk/news/2022/12/01/uk-face-prolonged-period-excess-deaths-following-pandemic-say. Accessed 2/2/2025

Ronan, P. (2022) Directives and Politeness in SPICE-Ireland. *Corpus Pragmatics* **6** (2), 175–199.

Rosoux, V. (2020) The role of memory in the desecuritization of inter-social conflicts. In: Butler, M. J. (ed.) *Securitization Revisited: Contemporary Applications and Insights*. Routledge, Milton, pp. 194–216.

Roth, K. & Wengeler, M. (eds.) (2020) Corona. Essayistische Notizen zum Diskurs. *Aptum, Zeitschrift für Sprachkritik und Sprachkultur* **16** (2+3).

Rowling, J. K. (1999) *Harry Potter and the Sorcerer's Stone*. New York, NY, Scholastic.

Rubin, O. & Baekkeskov, E. (2020) Expert-Led Securitization: The Case of the 2009 Pandemic in Denmark and Sweden. *Politics and Governance* **8** (4), 319–330.

Rutledge, P. E. (2020) Trump, COVID-19, and the War on Expertise. *The American Review of Public Administration* **50** (6–7), 505–511.

Rychnovská, D. (2014) Securitization and the Power of Threat Framing. *Perspectives* **22** (2), 9–31.

Salayo, J. (2020) Social Distancing, Community Quarantine and Bullets: A Critical Discourse Analysis of Pres. Rodrigo Duterte's Speeches on the War against COVID-19 Pandemic. *Middle Eastern Journal of Research in Education and Social Sciences* **1** (2), 233–256.

Saldaña, J. (2013) *The coding manual for qualitative researchers*, 2. ed. Sage; SAGE Publ, London and New York.

Samaniego Sánchez, A., Cárdenas Arguedas, S. & Lemus Muñiz, D. (2023) Mexico's Governmental Communication Strategy "Las Vespertinas" in Times of COVID-19: Crises and Strategies of a Populist Government. In: Musiał-Karg, M. & Luengo, Ó. G. (eds.) *Digital Communication and Populism in Times of Covid-19: Cases, Strategies, Examples*, 1st ed. 2023. Springer Nature Switzerland; Imprint Springer, Cham, pp 81–105.

Sanaa, I. & Kushi, Q. (2012) Facebook Status Updates: A Speech Act Analysis. *Academic Research International* **3** (2), 500–507.

Sanders, K. B. (2020) British government communication during the 2020 COVID-19 pandemic: Learning from high reliability organizations. *Church, Communication and Culture* **5** (3), 356–377.

Sari, D. & Utomo, A. (2020) Directive speech act in President Joko Widodo's speech related to handling coronavirus (Covid-19) in Indonesia (Pragmatic review). *Journal of Social Studies (JSS)* **16** (1), 35–50.

Sartika, D. & Irawan, A. M. (2021) Directive Speech Acts of Harry Potter, Ronald Weasley, and Hermione Granger in "Harry Potter and The Philosophers Stone" Movie Script. *English Language and Literature* **10** (4), 419.

Schotthöfer, A. (2024) Individuals in Securitization: Explaining US Presidents' Choice to (De)Securitize North Korea. *Foreign Policy Analysis* **20** (3), 1–21.

Schueler, D. & Marx, M. (2023) Speech acts in the Dutch COVID-19 Press Conferences. *Language resources and evaluation* **57** (2), 869–892.

Seale, H., Harris-Roxas, B., Heywood, A., Abdi, I., Mahimbo, A., Chauhan, A. & Woodland, L. (2022) Speaking COVID-19: supporting COVID-19 communication and engagement efforts with people from culturally and linguistically diverse communities. *BMC public health* **22** (1), 1257.

Seargeant, P. (2023) *Crisis Leadership: Boris Johnson and Political Persuasion during the Covid Pandemic*. Cambridge University Press, Cambridge.

Searle, J. R. (1969) *Speech acts*. Cambridge, Cambridge University Press.

Searle, J. R. (1976) A Classification of Illocutionary Acts. *Language in Society* **5** (1), 1–23.

Searle, J. R. (1977) Reiterating the Differences: A Reply to Derrida. *Glyph* 2.

Searle, J. R. (2012 [1979]) *Expression and meaning. Studies in the theory of speech acts.* Cambridge, Cambridge Univ. Press.

Semino, E. (2021) "Not Soldiers but Fire-fighters": Metaphors and Covid-19. *Health communication* **36** (1), 50–58.

Seok, S., Hwang, E., Choi, J. & Lim, Y. (2022) Cultural Differences in Indirect Speech Act Use and Politeness in Human-Robot Interaction. In: *17th ACM/IEEE International Conference on Human-Robot Interaction (HRI)*, pp. 1–8.

Serrano-Contreras, I.-J. & Díaz-Montiel, A. (2023) Feminist Framing in Times of Pandemic: An Analysis of the Spanish Case. In: Musiał-Karg, M. & Luengo, Ó. G. (eds.) *Digital Communication and Populism in Times of Covid-19: Cases, Strategies, Examples*. Springer Nature Switzerland, Cham, pp. 29–40.

Seufert, A., Poignée, F., Hoßfeld, T. & Seufert, M. (2022) Pandemic in the digital age: analyzing WhatsApp communication behavior before, during, and after the COVID-19 lockdown. *Humanities and Social Sciences Communications* **9** (1).

Shepherd, J., Harris, B., Murphy, R. & Vizard, T. (2023) *Public opinions and social trends, Great Britain: Coronavirus (COVID-19) and other illnesses, 22 March to 2 April 2023*. Office for National Statistics. Available at: https://www.ons.gov.uk/peoplepopulationandcommunity/wellbeing/datasets/publicopinionsandsocialtrendsgreatbritaincoronaviruscovid19andotherillnesses/. Accessed 01/07/2025.

Shkvorchenko, N., Hromovenko, V. & Sharapanovska, Y. (2021) The concept of "pandemic" in modern English-language political discourse. *Revista Amazonia Investiga* **10** (46), 225–233.

Short, M. (2007) How to Make a Drama out of a Speech Act: The Speech Act of Apology in the Film *A Fish Called Wanda*. *Stylistics* **3**, 169–189.

Sifianou, M. (2012) Disagreements, face and politeness. *Journal of Pragmatics* **44** (12), 1554–1564.

Silaški, N. & Đurović, T. (2022) From an invisible enemy to a football match with the virus: Adjusting the Covid-19 pandemic metaphors to political agendas in Serbian public discourse. In: Musolff, A., Breeze, R., Kondo, K. et al. (eds.). *Pandemic and crisis discourse*. Communicating COVID-19 and public health strategy. London, England, Bloomsbury, pp. 271–284.

Sinclair, J. (2004) *Trust the Text*. London, Routledge.

Sinclair, J. (2005) Meaning in the Framework of Corpus Linguistics. *Lexicographica* **20**, 20–32.

Sjöstedt, R. (2020) Assessing securitization theory: Theoretical discussions and empirical developments. In: Butler, M. J. (ed.) *Securitization Revisited: Contemporary Applications and Insights*. Routledge, Milton, pp. 28–46.

Sjöstedt, R., Kovacs, M. S. & Themnér, A. (2019) Demagogues of hate or shepherds of peace? Examining the threat construction processes of warlord democrats in Sierra Leone and Liberia. *Journal of International Relations and Development* **22** (3), 560–583.

Skinner, G. & Garrett, C. (2021) Number of people completely following COVID-19 restrictions falls, especially among 55–75-year olds. Available at: https://www.ipsos.com/en-uk/number-people-completely-following-covid-19-restrictions-falls-especially-among-55-75-year-olds. Accessed 03/03/2025.

Sodipo, O. (2021) Coronavirus disease pandemic and the securitization of migration in South Africa. *Journal of African Transformation* **6** (1), 141–160.

Sonderling, S. (2023) Covid-19 Pandemic: The role of non-metaphorical war metaphors and agonistic speech acts in constructing a post-democratic South Africa **15** (1), 127–166.

Soomro, A. & Aqdas, S. (2023) Research In Im/Politeness Across Cultures And Contexts. *Journal of Academic Research for Humanities* **3** (3), 122–129.

Sornbanlang, S. (2022) The Securitization of the Coronavirus in Asian Countries: A Paradox of National Security and Human Security During the COVID-19 Crisis. In: Varin, C. (ed.) *Global Security in Times of Covid-19*. Springer International, Cham, pp. 145–170.

Spring Research Team (2022) The COVID-19 third wave in Myanmar following the military coup. *F1000Research* **11**, 1301.

Spyridonidis, D., Côté, N., Currie, G. & Denis, J.-L. (2022) Leadership configuration in crises: Lessons from the English response to COVID-19. *Leadership* **18** (5), 680–694.

Stefanowitsch, A. (2020) *Corpus linguistics: A guide to the methodology*. Berlin, Language Science Press.

Stewart, H. (2020) 'Beacon of light': Capt Tom Moore to be knighted. *The Guardian,* May 19. Available at: https://www.theguardian.com/world/2020/may/19/beacon-of-light-capt-tom-moore-to-be-knighted. Accessed 09/09/2024.

Stivas, D. & Sliwinski, K. (2023) The securitization of the COVID-19 pandemic in Europe, Asia, and Oceania: Mixes of imbalanced securitizing narratives and measures. *Stosunki Międzynarodowe – International Relations* **3**, 16.

Stivas, D. (2023) Greece's response to the European refugee crisis: A tale of two securitizations. *Mediterranean Politics* **28** (1), 49–72.

Streeck, J. (1980) Speech acts in interaction: A critique of Searle. *Discourse Processes* **3** (2), 133–153.

Stritzel, H. (2014) *Security in Translation*. London, Palgrave Macmillan.

Subramanian, S., Cohn, T. & Baldwin, T. (2019) Target Based Speech Act Classification in Political Campaign Text. In: *Proceedings of the eighth joint conference on lexical and computational semantics*, pp. 273–282.

Sumaila, U. R., Cisneros-Montemayor, A. M. & Dyck, A. et al. (2012) Impact of the Deepwater Horizon well blowout on the economics of US Gulf fisheries. *Canadian Journal of Fisheries and Aquatic Sciences* **69** (3), 499–510.

Surová, S. (2022) Securitization and militarized quarantine of Roma settlements during the first wave of COVID-19 pandemic in Slovakia. *Citizenship Studies* **26** (8), 1032–1062.

Tanduk, R. (2023) Pragmatic Aspects of Speech Acts: A Cross-Linguistic Perspective. *English Review: Journal of English Education* **11** (3), 881–890.

Taylor, C. (2013) Searching for similarity using corpus-assisted discourse studies. *Corpora* **8** (1), 81–113.

Taylor, C. (2014) Investigating the representation of migrants in the UK and Italian press. *International Journal of Corpus Linguistics* **19** (3), 368–400.

The Guardian (2020) PM's Covid-19 timeline: From 'mild symptoms' to a brush with death. *The Guardian,* April 12. Available at: https://www.theguardian.com/world/2020/apr/05/timeline-boris-johnson-and-coronavirus. Accessed 09/09/2024.

Thorne, T. (2020) #CORONASPEAK. The Language of Covid-19 Goes Viral. *Language and Innovation, Blog*. Available at: https://language-and-innovation.com/2020/03/31/coronaspeak-the-language-of-covid-19-goes-viral/. Accessed 2/2/2025.

Tirthali, D. & Murai, Y. (2024) Facilitating open online discussions: speech acts inspiring and hindering deep conversations. *Open Learning: The Journal of Open, Distance and e-Learning* **39** (3), 280–296.

Tomkins, L. (2020) Where is Boris Johnson? When and why it matters that leaders show up in a crisis. *Leadership* **16** (3), 331–342.

Tomlinson, S. (2026) *Education and race from empire to multiracial Britain*, 2nd edition. Policy Press, Bristol.

Törenli, N. & Kıyan, Z. (2023) The Importance of Sustainable Communication in the Covid-19 Period: The Case of Turkey. In: Servaes, J. & Yusha'u, M. J. (eds.) *SDG18 Communication for All, Volume 2*. Springer International, Cham, pp. 225–246.

Trombetta, M. (ed.) (2023) *Handbook on climate change and international security*. Edward Elgar, Cheltenham, UK.

UK Parliament (2024) Question Time. Available at: https://www.parliament.uk/about/how/business/questions/. Accessed 1/2/2025.

Vankovska, B. (2020) Dealing with COVID-19 in the European periphery: between securitization and "gaslighting". *Journal of Global Faultlines* **7** (1), 71–88.

Ventura, S. (2022) The Italian Government's Pandemic Communication from Giuseppe Conte to Mario Draghi: Between "Leadership Building" and "Crisis Resolution". In: Maarek, P. J. (ed.) *Manufacturing Government Communication on Covid-19*. Springer International, Cham, pp. 253–271.

Verbi (2024a) MAXQDA: MAXQDA Analytics Pro. [Software]. Version 24.4.1. Berlin, Germany: VERBI Software.

Verbi (2024b) Document Comparison Chart: A Visual Comparison of Coded Text. *MAXQDA*. Available at: https://www.maxqda.com/help-mx22/visual-tools/document-comparison-chart-a-visual-comparison-of-coded-text. Accessed 09/12/2024.

Vessey, R. (2023) Language and gender in Canadian Chief Medical Officers' tweets during the COVID-19 pandemic. *Critical Discourse Studies* **20** (2), 200–217.

Vizard, T. (2020) *Coronavirus and the social impacts on Great Britain: 11 December 2020.: Opinions and Lifestyle Survey (COVID-19 module), 2 to 6 December*. Office for National Statistics, Available at: www.ons.gov.uk. https://www.ons.gov.uk/file?uri=/peoplepopulationandcommunity/healthandsocialcare/healthandwellbeing/datasets/coronavirusandthesocialimpactsongreatbritaindata/current/previous/v37/referencetables1112201012202017O525.xlsx. Accessed 01/07/2025.

Vogler, A. (2023) Tracking Climate Securitization: Framings of Climate Security by Civil and Defense Ministries. *International Studies Review* **25** (2), 1–27.

Vuori, J. A. (2008) Illocutionary Logic and Strands of Securitization: Applying the Theory of Securitization to the Study of Non-Democratic Political Orders. *European Journal of International Relations* **14** (1), 65–99.

Vuori, J. A. (2025) Securitization as a context-changing speech act. *Cooperation and Conflict* **60** (4), 1054–1072.

Wæver, O. & Buzan, B. (2020) Racism and responsibility – The critical limits of deepfake methodology in security studies: A reply to Howell and Richter-Montpetit. *Security Dialogue* **51** (4), 386–394.

Wæver, O., Buzan, B., Kelstrup, M. & Lemaitre, P. (1993) *Identity, Migration and the New Security Order in Europe*. London, Pinter.

Walker, P. (2021) Keep life moving: The latest in a long line of UK Covid mantras. *The Guardian*, July 21. Available at: https://www.theguardian.com/world/2021/jul/21/keep-life-moving-the-latest-in-a-long-line-of-uk-covid-mantras. Accessed 09/09/2024.

Walker, P., Sabbagh, D. & Syal, R. (2020) Boris Johnson boots out top adviser Dominic Cummings. *The Guardian*, November 13. Available at: https://www.theguardian.com/politics/2020/nov/13/dominic-cummings-has-already-left-job-at-no-10-reports. Accessed 10/10/2024.

Wallaschek, S. & Ziegler, F. (2021) Making sense of the 'new normal': The COVID-19 crisis in the communication of the prime ministers of Ireland and New Zealand. *Culture, Practice & Europeanization* **6** (1), 112–134.

Wang, K.-C. (2021) Securitization of Public Policy and Pandemic: Taiwan's Case Against Covid-19. *WIMAYA* **2** (1), 1–7.

Wang, X., Kaur, S., Mat Isa, N. & Kaur, S. (2024) Image restoration strategies in pandemic crisis communication: a comparative analysis of Chinese and American COVID-19 political speeches. *Humanities and Social Sciences Communications* **11** (1).

Warner, J. & Boas, I. (2019) Securitization of climate change: How invoking global dangers for instrumental ends can backfire. *Environment and Planning C: Politics and Space* **37** (8), 1471–1488.

Wasserman, H. & Madrid-Morales, D. (2022) The Messenger, the Message, and the Receiver: South African Government Communication During the COVID-19 Pandemic. In: Maarek, P. J. (ed.) *Manufacturing Government Communication on Covid-19*. Springer International, Cham, pp. 319–333.

Weiss, G. & Wodak, R. (eds.) (2003) *Critical discourse analysis*. Theory and interdisciplinarity. Basingstoke, Palgrave Macmillan.

Weisser, M. (2015) *Practical corpus linguistics*. An introduction to corpus-based language analysis. Chichester, West Sussex, UK, Wiley-Blackwell.

Wicke, P. & Bolognesi, M. (2020) Framing COVID-19: How we conceptualize and discuss the pandemic on Twitter. *PloS one* **15** (9), e0240010.

Wik, T. & Neal, A. (2024) The prioritisation of climate security: A content analysis of national security agendas. *Environment and Security* **3** (1), 33–71.

Wilhelmsen, J. (2017) *Russia's securitization of Chechnya: How war became acceptable*. Routledge, London, New York, NY.

Wilkinson, C. (2007) The Copenhagen School on Tour in Kyrgyzstan: Is Securitization Theory Useable Outside Europe? *Security Dialogue* **38** (1), 5–25.

Winiarska-Brodowska, M. (2022) COVID-19 and Government Communication in Poland. In: Maarek, P. J. (ed.) *Manufacturing Government Communication on Covid-19*. Cham, Springer International, pp. 335–352.

Wodak, R. & Meyer, M. (eds.) (2016) Methods of Critical Discourse. London, Sage.

World Health Organization (2023) COVAX: Working for global equitable access to COVID-19 vaccines. Available at: https://www.who.int/initiatives/act-accelerator/covax. Accessed 09/09/2024.

Wynne, M. (2008) Searching and concordancing. In: Lüdeling, A. & Kytö, M. (eds.) *Corpus Linguistics: An international handbook*. Berlin, de Gruyter, pp. 706–737.

Xue, J., Chen, J., Chen, C., Zheng, C., Li, S. & Zhu, T. (2020) Public discourse and sentiment during the COVID 19 pandemic: Using Latent Dirichlet Allocation for topic modeling on Twitter. *PloS one* **15** (9), e0239441.

Yang, H. (2022) 'We are at war': securitisation, legitimation and COVID-19 pandemic politics in France. *Contemporary Politics* **29** (2), 207–227.

Yasin, H., Mansoor, F. & Thalho, N. (2021) A critical discourse analysis of a public service speech by PM Imran Khan. *Journal of Archaeology of Egypt/Egyptology* **18** (7), 2824–2834.

Young, S. (2022) Rituals, Reassurance, and Compliance: Government Communication in Australia during the COVID-19 Pandemic. In: Maarek, P. (ed.) *Manufacturing Government Communication on Covid-19*. Springer International, Cham, pp. 147–174.

Yu, Y., Tay, D. & Yue, Q. (2023) Media representations of China amid COVID-19: A corpus-assisted critical discourse analysis. *Media International Australia* **191** (1), 73–87.

Zagidullina, M. V., Ghodrati, A. & Shafaghi, M. (2023) Linguacultural aspects of the value and semantic attitude to the speech act of promise in Russian. *Russian Journal of Linguistics* **27** (2), 418–443.

Zappavigna, M. & Dreyfus, S. (2022) "In these pandemic times": The role of temporal meanings in ambient affiliation about COVID-19 on Twitter. *Discourse, Context & Media* **47**, 100595.

Zielinski, M., Cowell, M., Bull, C., Veluvolu, M., Behne, M., Nowotny, K., Brinkley-Rubinstein, L. (2022) Policy and public communication methods among U.S. state prisons during the first year of the COVID-19 pandemic. *Health & justice* **10** (1), 27.

Appendix

Table A1: Stop list of excluded words within the 100 most frequent words in the corpus, including their rank in the original frequency list and their absolute frequency; sorted by rank

Rank	Word	Frequ. (abs.)	Rank	Word	Frequ. (abs.)	Rank	Word	Frequ. (abs.)
1	the	3078	28	now	279	65	which	112
2	and	2332	29	but	266	67	many	108
3	to	2168	30	not	249	69	one	108
5	of	1410	31	at	244	70	because	107
6	that	1017	33	if	219	72	over	105
7	in	997	34	by	218	76	when	99
8	a	731	37	who	194	81	about	94
14	this	561	42	these	166	83	first	92
15	for	544	43	those	161	89	some	89
17	as	444	46	out	150	90	where	89
20	on	409	48	or	140	91	how	88
21	with	374	49	there	140	94	across	86
23	so	337	55	also	124	96	an	84
26	from	292	62	than	114			
27	all	283	63	up	113			

Table A2: List of individual speech acts in the JPanC20; sorted by absolute frequency; speech acts with an equal number of occurrences sorted alphabetically

Rank	Speech act	Freq.		Rank	Speech act	Freq.
1	explain	119		26	advise	18
2	acknowledge others	88		27	praise others	18
3	promise	68		28	motivate	17
4	warn	53		29	impose rules	16
5	rely on science	49		30	give examples	15
6	issue a new policy	47		31	express anger	14
7	express confidence	45		32	implore	14
8	state	45		33	instruct	14
9	show understanding	44		34	praise himself / government	12
10	express caution	43		35	express hope	11
11	command	43		36	imply	11
12	report	43		37	express regret	11
13	thank	43		38	hedging/deflecting	10
14	calm/reassure	39		39	lift measures	9
15	boast/express pride	34		40	request	8
16	affirm	31		41	express relief	7
17	affirm prior policy	29		42	apologise	5
18	sympathise	27		43	express grief	5
19	declare something	26		44	personal experience	4
20	ask you to	25		45	express impatience	3
21	update	23		46	vow	2
22	commit himself to do sth	21		47	offer	1
23	describe	20		48	prohibit	1
24	narrate	20		49	threaten	1
25	answer	19				

Figure A1: Visualisation of speech act system

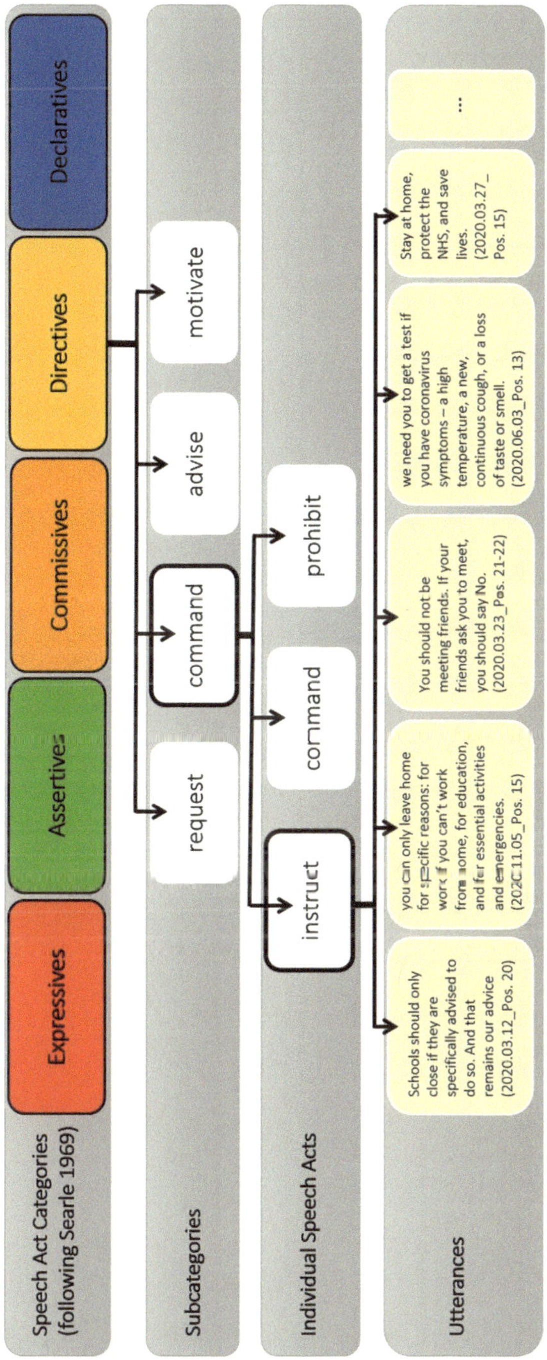

Figure A2: Speech act coverage in the JPanC20 by category, measured in characters; y-axis: number of characters including spaces; x-axis: number of individual speech acts within each category, sorted by relative frequency; categories coded by colour: red: expressives, green: assertives, orange: commissives, yellow: directives, blue: declaratives

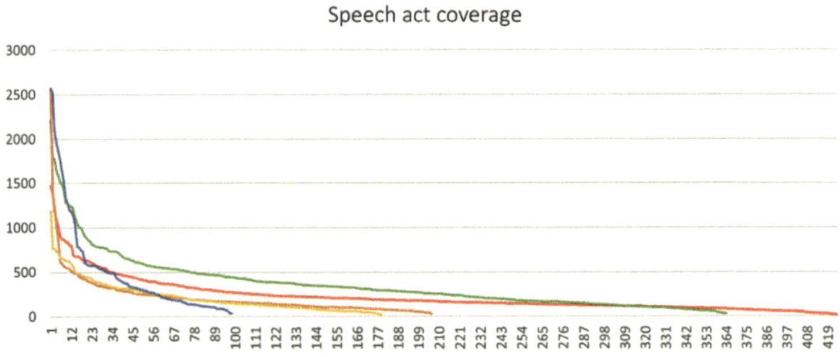

Table A1: Overview of speech act coverage extreme values and averages per category, measured in characters including spaces; values of averages rounded to the nearest decimal

	Expres-sives	Assertives	Commis-sives	Directives	Declara-tives
Number of speech acts	424	364	206	179	98
Maximum	1398	2210	2568	1187	2568
Minimum	13	30	29	20	32
Average	219,90	362,73	219,00	224,00	493,00